When the Cook Can't Look

WHEN THE COOK CAN'T LOOK

A Cooking Handbook for the Blind and Visually Impaired

Ralph Read

CONTINUUM · New York

1981
The Continuum Publishing Corporation
18 East 41st Street, New York, N.Y. 10017

Printed in the United States of America

Library of Congress Cataloging in Publication Data

Read, Ralph R
When the cook can't look.
1. Cookery for the blind. I. Title.
TX652.R373 641.5'02408161 80–25629
ISBN 0–8264–0034–5

For Tom Albright,
who yelled at the right time

These people helped me greatly
in planning and writing this book.
I am deeply grateful to them:

Skip and Skippy Acuff, Tom Albright,
Edna Brown, Mark and Angela Gretchen,
Vivian Ivey, Robert and Joyce Lehmeyer,
Richard Mills, Hans-Bernhard Moeller,
Gene and Mikey Read, Dennis Samford,
Marion Wilson, A. Leslie Willson,
and Rick Nicholas.

Contents

Part One

BECOMING A COOK

Why the Blind Should Cook

Cookbooks exist in virtually every imaginable category, up to and including voluminous sets with which ambitious gourmets can cook their way from country to country around the entire globe. An average home may have more than a dozen cookbooks. There are avid collectors who own literally hundreds. But for the blind people in this country no good cookbook exists. Is there a use for one? You ask in surprise. What is a blind person doing trying to cook anyway?

There is not only a use but also a need for such a cookbook. Three good reasons come to mind immediately:

1. *Practicality.* Whether blind people live alone or with family or friends, they should be able to cope in the kitchen, at least in a modest way. And this book will teach them how to cope in more than just a modest way. The greater the normalcy that can be restored to the lives of the blind, the less obtrusive is the handicap.

People tend to smother the handicapped with kindness. As a blind friend of yours moves toward the kitchen, I can hear you rising to your feet with an automatic "Here, let me do that." For in the dark, surely the kitchen is nothing but an arsenal of booby traps, of things that smash and cut and burn. Nonsense. The secret is all in technique. That is, how to do without eyes the things that seem so simple with vision. You can test any of the procedures, the techniques suggested in this book, simply by trying them out with your eyes shut. Just remember: the difference between you and the cooks this book has been written for is that you can peek, and they can't.

2. *Pride.* In addition to the great practical advantage of restored independence, there is the element of pride. This is an intangible which I believe cannot be underestimated. The more the blind can do by themselves, the less the doldrums and depression will creep into their lives and the specter of self-pity will no longer be feared. I remember the pride I felt when I finally successfully invented a method of frying my eggs "easy over," the way I like them best. I felt as proud as if I had just been graduated as a Cordon Bleu Chef, and every bit as skillful.

3. *Enjoyment.* The fun of cooking ranges all the way from mere puttering—like making up a plate of snacks or improving on that boxed cake mix—to spending hours on creating a masterpiece that is as beautiful as it is delectable. The hobby of cooking is one that the blind too can enjoy. Here's hoping they'll quickly discover this.

This book is designed for people whose handicaps range from severe visual impairment of whatever kind to actual legal blindness to total and congenital blindness.

How to Use This Book

This book is meant to be read aloud, and with it you-the-reader will be able to observe and guide your novice cook step-by-step.

The "you" in the first three chapters of Part One refers to you-the-reader, not to the listener, whether you-the-reader are a friend or relative of the listener or simply someone looking at this book out of curiosity. In the "Techniques" chapter and in "Food Preparations" (Part Two), the "you" refers to you-the-listener or you-the-cook. You-the-cook will find it easiest to master the techniques by trying them out as your sighted assistant reads them aloud to you. You will thus be performing a cooking lesson together. Later on, you will need no assistance and will not need to wait until someone is at hand except to refresh your memory.

Since basic techniques are so important, from now on I will discard the word "recipes" and call them "food preparations" instead. This is to emphasize that the how-to-do-it in blind cookery is much more than a list of ingredients in their proper amounts. In fact, we can say that the most important ingredient *is* technique.

Refrain from jumping ahead into the food preparations. If you do, you will miss the introduction to the techniques. Technique is the central concept of the food preparations, and individual techniques are used in each one.

You-the-reader should first read all of Part One to yourself. When you begin to read to your listener, you can omit as much as you want, perhaps reading only the brief comments on reasons for the blind to cook in the preceding chapter. Then proceed to the techniques.

Read as many as you have time for at your first lesson, guiding your novice cook step-by-step. Then turn to the list of things that the cook can now do ("You Already Can"), that is, things the cook can do merely by learning those techniques, without even turning to the actual food preparations. Once many of the techniques are explained and tried out, they become reduced to nothing much more than common sense ("Why didn't I think of that?"), and the actual text of this part of the book may not need to be repeated.

Then turn to some Level 1 or 2 preparations—avoid the 3s at first—and choose a few of the most useful breakfast and lunch preparations. These will give your cook confidence and familiarity with the kitchen. The preparations are grouped according to levels of increasing difficulty, Level 1, 2, and 3, in the Appendix on p. 111.

The food preparations do not begin with a list of ingredients as most recipes do. It is difficult and impractical for a blind cook to memorize such a list out of context, particularly when he or she cannot easily refer to it again. Instead, each ingredient is introduced in its logical sequence as the techniques dictate. Any unusual or unexpected ingredients, however, are mentioned at the beginning of the preparation. There are no exotic ingredients in this cookbook. In fact, not a single one that cannot be bought at an ordinary, medium-sized supermarket in any American city.

Since there is no food store, not even a small one, within easy walking distance of my home, I necessarily ride to a supermarket with a friend. I do not enjoy shopping, so efficiency is at the top of my list. I try to do one major shopping per month buying staples, canned goods and meats that I can freeze. On small weekly trips I then pick up milk, fresh fruit and vegetables, and any items I will need for a special food preparation.

I type up my monthly grocery list, trying to be as complete as possible. I give the size, amount, quality and sometimes even the brand of items I want. I tag along through the store to facilitate any decision-making that is necessary, instead of waiting in the car. Besides, I have to sign the check when it's all added up.

I compile the monthly list by thinking in categories. First, what all the standard things are I use for breakfasts and lunches, and the staples I use in preparing dinner. Then—and this part of making the list is enjoyable—I try to target at least half a dozen dinner preparations for the next month that I particularly like or have not fixed for some time. Or that are new.

As cooks try out the preparations and move on to Level 3, they will undoubtedly be tempted to experiment with various techniques. They should feel free to go ahead and do so, but only if they are dissatisfied with the way I advise them to proceed, and then only if they are sure what they are trying out is perfectly safe. Certain personal modifications of techniques are inevitable.

As cooks gain in skill and confidence, they will be able to graft their knowledge of techniques onto recipes found in many ordinary cookbooks. They may find it possible to move on to recipes for things like soufflés and tempura vegetables which are too difficult to be called Level 3 preparations. Hence, they may even become Level 4 chefs.

You who are able to read may find yourself caught up in trying to understand the problems of the blind better, so I have included some incidental and anecdotal material about blindness that may not pertain directly to coping in the kitchen.

For the Sighted Reader

The first landmarks were concrete. They could be seen and felt. Early maps, highly imaginative as they were, nevertheless limited physical delineation to tangible features of oceans, lakes, rivers, and mountains. Legal property lines were drawn between boulders and hills, rivers and forests. Not until the late Middle Ages did the astrolabe permit navigators to measure latitudinal distances abstractly. Indeed, your county has now been surveyed and recorded down to the last square meter of its surface. But when you are driving a car, you are probably as dependent on proceeding from one familiar physical landmark to another as were early hunters and nomads in search of their livelihood.

The same is true of the blind, even though the graphic element of vision is omitted. True, I like to carry an abstract view of an area in my head, like a blueprint, but the features on the blueprint are all locatable by touch or hearing. No, I do not have any sixth sense. I do not have any radar or sonar. I do not even count steps. And yes, I do bump into things. If it were not for my "long cane," I would bump into even more things.

It is mostly a matter of landmarks. In an urban setting, these are few in kind and relatively easy to deal with.

To a blind person, a town is made up of stripes. Outside, these stripes are sidewalks and streets. Inside, they are hallways. In both instances, the stripes are punctuated by walls and doorways. Not a very colorful way of thinking of your surroundings, but practical when you are trying to get around. I add the trees and flowers and birds and people when I have a chance to sit down. The techniques one is taught for using the long cane enable one to maneuver corners, curbs, and miscellaneous obstacles, but above all, doors and steps.

Here is where the generosity and kindness of you sighted people can be a hindrance rather than a help. Most trained and experienced blind people do not need, and often do not want, help with doors and stairs. Of course, if I have my free arm full—that is, the one not wielding the cane—I welcome your help. Or if you spot a blind person handicapped in some other way, help him or her. But on the university campus, an environment familiar to me, when an eager student leaps out of the dark, yanks a door open in front of me, and happily proclaims "The door is open!", I can only smile and thank him. How curmudgeonly it would be for me to stop and lecture him, letting him know that he has deprived me of a useful landmark. I would only have made both of us late for class.

Steps too can be a problem. I know where they are supposed to be along my route. I know how to start up the stairs and how to start down them. I approach them slowly because that is the way to do it. This or that student will swoop up from behind and grab me enthusiastically by the shoulder. On several memorable occasions I have almost been shoved down the stairs.

Be as friendly as you always have been. Just ask: "Can I help you?" first. Often you can; often I want you to. And I always will thank you.

People ask whether my hearing has improved since I lost my eyesight. Yes, but only in the sense that a blind person makes better use of the hearing he has to compensate for the vision he lacks. You do not have to worry about interfering with whatever sound signals I use to get my bearing. You won't throw me off course unless you jam that transistor radio of yours into my ear.

The remaining two senses are of little use in navigating. Only rarely can I employ the olfactory organ. For example, a large trash can is posted just where I often make a right turn into an office building on campus. If this receptacle has been ripening in the hot sun for most of the day, I can smell it from two or three yards away.

When I am walking with a friend or student, I give them the following simple rules for their role as a "sighted guide":

1. Never tug at me (unless you are yanking me out of the path of disaster). This common mistake only tends to pull me off balance, and it places your back to traffic and obstacles of all sorts, effectively rendering you blind too.

2. Instead, lead me. Since I am right-handed, I will grasp your right arm above the elbow with my left hand. (If I were left-handed, I would take your left arm with my right hand.) I will follow you about half a stride behind.

3. Give me a brief running commentary on obstacles: "Curb coming up . . . It's kind of bumpy here . . . and so on." Walk through doors ahead of me, telling me what kind of door we are encountering: "Door opens out, to the left", or "Door opens in, to the right", and so on. If I am carrying my long cane in my right hand, instead of sweeping with it I will hold it several inches above the ground about a foot and a half directly in front of me to help locate obstacles.

4. When climbing or descending stairs, go one step ahead of me. This helps me keep my balance, as well as letting me judge the height of each step and the pitch of the stairs.

5. It is natural to gesture when giving directions, so you need to remember that body English does nothing for me. "Right over there" is no help at all. Try to tell me whether I need to turn to my left or my right, and how far I have to go—a hundred yards, one block. If you notice any obvious obstacles, such as overhanging branches or a child's tricycle parked on the sidewalk, let me know about them.

On first encounter with me, some people unconsciously assume that I am deaf as well as blind, and even that I am feebleminded. This overreaction comes from their having had so little contact with the blind, and not knowing what to do or say.

Recently I went to vote in a local election, and the well-meaning but self-conscious voting judge was a case in point. Although I was within arm's length of her, she turned to ask the friend who had come along with me, "Can he sign his own name?" Then, after helping me vote, she said loudly and slowly to me, "Good, good," and patted me firmly and approvingly on the shoulder, as if praising a small child who had managed to perform a difficult task.

It is the initial encounter that makes other people nervous. Upon subsequent contact, they find it much easier to act themselves. Since my students see me from three to five times a week, they get used to the handicap in short order. In fact, they can even joke about it. One class in particular liked to distract me from the topic of German grammar, which was official class business, so I would ramble on about my personal experiences living in Europe. Once, in mock anger, I threw a piece of chalk at a clever student who had managed to do just that. And hit him, much to the delight of the other students. "How did you manage that?" he inquired, perplexed. "Blind luck," I shot back. The laughter that followed was almost an ovation.

For simplicity's sake, I will usually use the word "blind" in this book. The blind do not like their language censored, and you should not feel hesitant about using words like "see," "look," and "blind" in their company. As a matter of fact, I use them myself. "I'll see you tomorrow," is a common remark for me to make.

I hope those pointers will be useful for people who are first associating with the blind. It may also be useful to describe what may happen to people who are first encountering blindness. This is a *possible* emotional progression in the newly blind.

It is obvious that those who go blind during their lifetime have one enormous advantage over those who are born blind: experience and skill in forming visual concepts. My head is full of maps of familiar places. Put to use like a schematic drawing or a blueprint, they greatly improve both the confidence and speed of my mobility. The once-sighted person can usually learn new routes and assimilate patterns of movement in strange places more rapidly too, by visualizing the new map mentally. There are also the thousands of memories, of people, of things, of nature, that remain permanently as treasured mental photographs. Nevertheless, the trauma of *going* blind is something the congenitally blind do not suffer. The affliction of blindness can approach as swiftly as an automobile accident or as slowly as progressive glaucoma.

A possible progression of one's going blind is relatively easy to chart. What follows is a theoretical view. In any given case, a person's response may seem caught for a long time at one of these stages, or his or her attitude may suddenly deteriorate or improve. But here is a realistic look at what can happen:

1. *Rejection.* The shock of what has happened is simply too great to be absorbed all at once. The defensive reaction is "This can't be happening to me. It is all a mistake, a bad dream, it will go away—it is only temporary, a freak side effect, and the doctor will tell me that in a few days I'll have my vision back." This panicky stage does not last long, however, as the concrete actuality of what has happened refuses to be swept aside, and the doctors remind you that they are only doctors, not miracle workers, and that you must face your new handicap.

2. *Resentment.* The next stage in this irrational but all too comprehensible progression is one of resentment. Only now does one fully realize how much one has lost, and how much one had previously taken for granted. That it should happen to you is preposterous, and surely will wreck your life. This new thought (which itself is preposterous) casts you in the role of the unique sufferer. You are the first person to whom this has ever happened. Why has this impossible burden been placed on you, out of all the billions on earth? Your anger and resentment turn more and more into frustration as your mind comes to realize the truth of your condition. You still do not know how to face your problem, and thus are in a stage of reaction rather than action. Your handicap is in control of you instead of your being in control of your handicap.

3. *Depression.* This and the next two stages form a continuum, a sort of downward slide in which it is difficult to draw clear lines

between the phases. Newly blind should have professional aid from the very beginning. Not just family help and sympathy, but professional counseling and mobility training are absolute musts by this stage. By now, the difficulty in doing things is no longer a novelty which causes shock with each new and dismaying discovery, but a humdrum and everyday expectation that produces constant frustration. The victim—for that is still how the person perceives him or herself—grows more and more used to being waited on. The island of remaining independence is being slowly eroded by the well-meaning and indeed necessary help that is received from all sides. The person's power for ordinary tasks, indeed ordinary life patterns, diminishes. It is only natural that the self-pity which has been waiting for its chance finds it easily as depression deepens.

My own "rites of passage" afford a good example of how easily self-pity can creep in. I was sitting at the kitchen table, trying to take a vitamin pill. I opened the pill bottle and reached for a glass of water, which I did not knock over. Then I reached for the pills again, pushing the bottle onto the floor, and scattering about a hundred pills. As the tinkle of the bouncing, dancing pills reached my ears, I began to cry. I felt so miserably sorry for myself that for a moment I could feel nothing else. But as the sound of the pills subsided, I realized quickly enough how ludicrous the situation was. A grown man crying over spilt vitamin pills. The utter triviality of the incident served to put me on guard against self-pity at a time when I was most vulnerable to it. Those pills contributed to my well-being in an unpredictable way.

This stage too is nonproductive. But worse still, it can signify the beginning of the alienation of other people from the sufferer as well as the sufferer from him or herself. Grousing and grumping are only one step away from self-pity. Understanding rather than feeling sorry for "the poor guy" is called for now. Indeed, it may be time to repeat the hoary cliché about just-think-how-many-people-are-worse-off-than-you-are.

4. *Despair.* Attitudinal problems are often so irrational that the

descent into the slough of despair may be successfully interrupted anywhere along the way. This is only a pattern and nothing about it is inevitable. But it is with this phase that feeling sorry for oneself sets in in earnest, and the "victim" may not realize until it is too late that the quagmire has become quicksand. Constant depression and a sort of gloomy introspection, rethinking again and again the same "if only" thoughts, characterize this phase. The threat is equally great, however, as a forerunner of the thorough emotional paralysis to come.

5. *Defeat.* When the handicapped lose the desire to help themselves as well as the belief that they can be helped, they reach a static condition that can only be labeled defeat. Sadly enough, some of the blind simply give up. What ensues, a life of mere sitting, usually indoors, while staring off into the (unperceived) middle distance is hardly a life at all. If the fourth stage is a sort of ruminating, the fifth is one of vegetating. It is the end of hope and the end of joy. And it is wholly unnecessary.

Kitchen Inventories

These are basic items that you will need throughout this book, so now you can go over my checklists. If you are about to start cooking in an average home kitchen, you will probably find it equipped with virtually everything listed here. You will also find many more things that are not listed. If you are starting from scratch, rest assured that none of these items represents an unnecessary expense, or something you will use only once in a blue moon.

Utensils and Equipment Checklist:

- measuring cup with raised numbers
- measuring spoons
- slotted spoon
- ladle
- large cooking spoon
- wooden spoon (optional)
- serving spoon
- corkscrew (optional)
- serrated knife (steak knife)
- paring knife
- carving knife
- carving fork (optional)
- knife sharpener (optional, very rarely used)
- cheese grater
- garlic press (optional)
- sieve
- funnel
- paper napkins
- paper towels
- paper plates (optional)

wax paper
plastic bags
plastic glasses (optional, I use the free ones some drinks come in)
aluminum foil
spatula
wire whisk
wall can opener
bottle opener
hand can opener (church key)
potholders
oven mitts
pastry brush (optional)
tongs (optional)
jar wrench or rubber jar opener
hand-turned food mixer
onion chopper
vegetable peeler
vegetable steamer (optional)
large cutting board or breadboard
small cutting board
timer
slicing guide (optional)
egg separator (optional)
freezer storage containers
skewers (optional, for closing roast fowl)
quart jars (optional, for soaking things and refrigerator storage)
tea egg
standard tableware
mixing bowls

Herbs, Spices, Condiments Checklist:

sugar
brown sugar (optional)
molasses (optional)
honey
salt
black pepper (preferably coarse ground)
garlic powder
garlic salt
fresh garlic (optional)
oregano
marjoram
basil
Italian seasoning (optional)
bay leaves
tarragon (used in one recipe)
powdered yellow mustard
dried onion flakes
chili powder
cinnamon (optional, for rice pudding and hot cereal)
saccharin (optional)
beef and chicken bouillon cubes
Worcestershire sauce
cumin seed
paprika
dill weed (for yellow and red vegetables and stroganoff)

curry powder
nutmeg (optional)
thyme
vanilla
soy sauce
red wine vinegar
cheap red cooking wine
(optional)
parsley flakes
cloves (optional)
bread crumbs
ketchup
lemon juice

Pots, Pans Checklist:

You can make all the preparations in this book with the following pots, pans, and miscellany. Of course you may have many more.

cake pan (nonspecified)
glass pie dish
loaf pan
two cookie sheets
large iron skillet (10 x 3 with cover)
medium-size iron skillet (8-inch diameter)
little iron skillet (6½-inch diameter)
nonstick skillet (medium size)
two 2½-quart aluminum pans
two or three 3-cup aluminum sauce pans
double boiler (optional)
roasting pan (with cover and rack size of your choice)
miscellaneous pan lids
vegetable steamer
all-purpose oven pan (square 8 x 8 x 2)
at least three oven casserole dishes (1½–3 quarts)
baking dish (9 x 13 x 2)

Techniques

Introduction

Most cookbooks are a compendium of lists. Often there is no introduction to speak of. What the users want, and what they find, are the hundreds of formulas that present themselves column after column. The format is taken for granted: first a cataloguing of the ingredients in their proper amounts, then the necessary directions for their successful combination. The directions, usually written in stripped-down telegram style, take it for granted that the cook already is familiar with basic and not so basic techniques. Beginners often encounter cryptic passages in the directions that leave them at a loss. The recipes—to use the word for the last time—differ considerably from the food preparations to follow in Part Two, since it is the job of this book to concentrate on techniques and say the otherwise unsaid. Therefore an admonition: this section deals with basics to avoid the necessity of constant repetition in Part Two. Part Two introduces additional tips and techniques wherever they apply to a specific preparation.

Techniques in this section are graded Level 1, Level 2, and Level 3 in increasing order of difficulty. As you learn to manipulate materials and utensils with ease and confidence, I hope that some of you will graduate from these pages and proceed to the vast store of recipes awaiting you in other cookbooks.

Arranging

Getting ready. An eminent scholar once began a book with the sentence: "All other things equal, it is usually best to begin at the beginning." And so it is here: the beginning being the physical arrangements in which you will do your cooking, and probably much of your eating. I am thinking not so much of the layout of the kitchen, which can vary so greatly, but of the things kitchens inevitably have in common: cupboards, a counter, a table, a refrigerator and a stove. To make your beginning, you should decide where to place all your dishes, pots and pans, and utensils. Deciding where to keep staples, spices and condiments, and all other foodstuffs is important too, but at least with them you can call on your nose for help. Once these simple decisions are made, you will no longer have to worry about them, except as an occasional improvement suggests itself. The whole matter becomes a nonproblem.

It is curiously difficult to persuade people not to move things around in your kitchen, at least not without your foreknowledge and permission. You must convince them that you mean it, that the shift of a box from one shelf to another could cause a crisis in the midst of an otherwise routine operation. The only exception I can think of to this inviolable policy of nonrelocation is if someone is suddenly overpowered by the urge to wash some dirty dishes for you.

On a recent visit, my mother "tidied up" the kitchen a bit, as a result of which it took me an hour to find: 1) the coffee filters, 2) the coffee measure, and 3) the coffee itself, all of which had been left in plain view. You will find that if everything remains where you placed it, soon you will know where almost everything is down to the square inch. Here, then, are some guidelines.

Dishes. Stack or nest between waist and head level the dishes you use most. Here they are most secure and accessible. If you have to stretch and stand on tiptoe to reach a vessel, it is much more likely to fall victim to the fumble-and-grope syndrome, so place lesser used dishes up high. It is the common dishes like dinner or lunch plates, soup or cereal bowls, that you will reach for a dozen times a day. Larger and heavier dishes, such as platters and mixing bowls, store well below counters and in other places you have to stoop to reach. They have a shorter way to fall from there anyway.

Do not stack your dishes too ambitiously. You may have created a second Leaning Tower of Pisa without being aware of it. If you have the luxury of enough space, make only one row of stacks or nests per shelf. If you do not have to reach around behind them, you will again reduce breakage.

It is only normal for you to break more dishes than other people do. Many blind people drift into the habit of eating exclusively from plastic or paper plates, but I advise against this. Use them when you're in a hurry, like anyone else would, but don't get into a rut—it works against the principle of pride that is so important to the blind cook. No, of course you should not dine exclusively from Limoges and Rosenthal, but if you limit yourself to paper plates, you may in time follow this efficiency to its logical result and eat the plate too. It adds roughage to the diet.

Glasses. Glasses should be stored upside down for greater cleanliness and stability. If you must stack glasses to save space, avoid doing so when they are drying. This should prevent them from sticking. Remember that glasses are the most fragile and vulnerable items in your cupboard. How much fussing you want to do about glasses is largely a matter of personal choice. At one extreme, you can purchase a set of squat, splay-bottomed glasses; but it makes more sense to be philosophical about the occasional and inevitable casualties. You may want to use plastic glasses sometimes, since they are unbreakable and cheap. But they are light and easy to knock over. And they don't look nice enough for a company dinner.

This is an appropriate place to talk about handling glasses, wherever they are, but especially at table. If you have forgotten where you put down your glass, a collision and a mess may remind you. The two best ways of locating the glass are:

1. *Horizontal.* Slide one hand slowly about the tabletop until you make contact gently.

2. *Vertical.* Lower your hand repeatedly and slowly from a height of about one foot over the approximate area of the glass.

Both methods are safe and efficient, but the first is less conspicuous. Do not wave your hand around three or four inches above the table, as if you were simply trying to grasp the glass. Then you will surely knock it over.

The simple search operation is actually a kind of sweeping, and both the vertical and horizontal kinds of sweeping are quite useful when you are working at a counter or a table. Sweeping as a term is most often used to designate the principle in employing the long cane, and is thus the key to mobility for those blind people who use the long cane as their method of getting around. Sweeping with the long cane is a mobility technique that came into wide use after World War II, due largely to the many servicemen who lost their eyesight in war injuries.

Arranging is the key to finding. Remember if you arrange your kitchen functionally, you will soon know the location of every object in it down to the square inch. It is important for you to convince people that they must without fail return every object exactly to its former location. If they put it on the wrong shelf, they might just as well have left it in the grocery store for all the good it does you.

Cupboard. Memory and touch work together when you arrange your cupboard. There is even something called tactile memory: your hands may help you remember where something is by trying to touch it, or how something works by actually touching it. I keep boxes of things together, and cans together, but on different shelves. It is relatively easy to remember what shape box something was in. For instance, you can tell even an unopened cereal box from a cracker box by shaking and squeezing it. Cans are trickier. With the help of a sighted person you can initial them with raised letters made by a plastic tape marker if you need to, or tear some of the label off this can or that. I just arrange them alphabetically, from left to right or from front to back on the shelf: beans, corn, hash, peas. Soups are in their own group: mushroom, onion, vegetable. Some cans, like sardine or corned beef, have distinctive shapes.

You don't need to alphabetize bags of things, because you can just pinch them. Split peas do not feel like elbow macaroni.

Some herbs, spices, and condiments, such as Worcestershire sauce, have distinguishing containers; but many come in identical containers. You will have so many of them that alphabetizing might give you too long a list and an inacurrate count. So, just use your sense of smell.

Refrigerator. Not much special advice can be given you about arranging foods in the refrigerator; you are largely a victim of your refrigerator's size, like everyone else. Besides, most refrigerators are carefully designed according to where what should go inside them. You should pay special attention, though, to keeping opened containers and leftovers at the front of shelves. Otherwise you will probably forget about them in the back of the shelf, where in the course of a few weeks they will grow thick, furry strands of some new strain of antibiotic mold.

You can use some good advice about defrosting the refrigerator, if you do not have a frost-free one. Slow down; do not try to do a speed job with all or most of the food still in it, as so many people try to. Somewhere around the house you have a picnic cooler, be it merely one made of cheap styrofoam. Place all your frozen goods and everything that spoils quickly—milk, potato salad, and so forth—in the cooler to protect it. Then empty out the rest of the fridge, making sure to not forget the drawers at the bottom, so you will not care how much water drips down onto the shelves as the ice melts.

Now you can proceed with the classic, tedious method: place pans of hot water in the freezer, replenishing them with boiling water as they cool and do their job. In the meantime, you should be embarked on some other project, like listening to a good book because it may take three hours or longer to do the job well. Do not attack remaining chunks of ice with hammer, screwdriver, and butcher knife, as you dearly desire to: you are much more likely to puncture or break a coolant line than you realize and to injure yourself in the bargain. This is one of those lazyday chores.

Opening Containers

To protest that most of my suggestions boil down to nothing much more than common sense, might be true, but nothing is more uncommon than common sense. How many times have you wrestled with a problem, stymied, until someone took it away from you and solved it with a swift twist? "Oh," you said, feeling slightly foolish.

Cans. Four basic types are cut, punch, pull-top and key. The best way to learn or relearn how to use a wall can opener is to have someone demonstrate it several times, really using a can, while you feel along. But basically, most can openers work like this: you pull back a lever as far as it will go in order to open the gap between two wheels that must co-operate: a cutting wheel (the top one) and the gripping wheel (the bottom one). A little lower down, there is usually some sort of angle or brace protruding slightly, against which the can leans while it is turning. The point is to make sure that the lip of the can stays securely between the two wheels as you push the lever back into place, while the can is also snug against the lower metal brace. If you are successful, there will be an unmistakable "biting" feeling as the cutting wheel cuts through the metal and you begin to turn the handle. Don't let go of the can with your other hand as you crank the handle, though. At first you may have enough difficulty getting the hang of using a can opener that you'll grade it a Level 3 task, but it is really only a Level 2. Usually I can open a can on the first try, but sometimes for no apparent reason it will take me three or four. Remember, the great majority of cans still open this way, so it is definitely worth the bother to learn.

The old-fashioned, hand-held can opener still comes in handy on picnics and camping, so as a backup it is good to have one around. It is built on the same principle, but takes strong hands and wrists to operate—definitely a Level 3 utensil, about as much fun as lighting a fire by rubbing two sticks together. Keep the can resting on something; don't wave it around in the air.

Punching open a beverage can with a "church key": nothing to learn here; most sighted people could do it with their eyes closed.

Pull-top cans are a little more dangerous to open than the pop-top beverage cans, because the entire lid comes off, as a circle or a spiral. Be sure to keep the hand holding the can entirely below the rim of the can; a cut from that lid can be nasty. You may want to pry the ring up with a table knife or the bowl of a spoon to break the vacuum.

Few cans still use a key opener; even the coffee can gave it up years ago. About the only common key-opening cans nowadays contain corned beef, patented lunch meats, ham, and sardines. And most people don't even like sardines. The problem with the keys is that the coil of metal that winds around the key as you open the can so often collapses, leaving you with no leverage and a sharp, dangerous snarl of metal. By this time, however, you can usually pry the can open the rest of the way with a sturdy knife. This requires holding onto the sharp lid of the can with your other hand, which must be carefully protected by an oven mitt.

Jars. I recommend a jar wrench for stubborn jars; the dime store will have them. There are several kinds but the cheapest and most convenient is a rubber grip pad. You would be wise to avoid the violent measures customarily taken with recalcitrant jar lids. Whacking them with the handle of a table knife is only one. If you have that much trouble, let someone else do it.

Bottles. Whether they have resealable twist-off caps or pry-off caps, I always run my finger around the mouth of the bottle after opening, to make sure the glass has not cracked or a chip been dislodged.

Boxes. Boxes with a pour spout or simple flap top are standard and easy to handle. As for the rest of them, as my dad would say, you have a hunting license. Over the years some perverse souls in the packaging industry have been hard at work devising more and more intricate, puzzling, and pointless ways to open and shut boxes. They rival jigsaw puzzles in their complexity, and the directions for their operation were written by income tax specialists on their days off . . . punch, tear, fold back, crease, discard this tab, expose cutter edge. Either get someone else to do it for you or just use violence—it's only paper, after all. Secure the box afterward by using a rubber band, as I do. Some of the worst packages to open, curiously enough, seem to be those which in turn contain more packaging: plastic and aluminum wraps of various kinds.

You will probably find that rolls of plastic or cellophane wrap that cling are the worst of all to use, for once the wrap starts sticking to itself on the roll, which it invariably does, it is very difficult to pull apart again without being able to see it. Try turning back the clock and using waxed paper and rubber bands. It will improve your blood pressure.

Pouring

That you can pour liquids accurately and without spilling will be a pleasant surprise to you. Of greatest help is the *dipstick* technique, which simply means having an index finger at the right place at the right time. Hold your glass securely at the very top by encircling it with your hand; make sure the glass is resting on a firm surface. Put your index finger inside the glass, with the top as far down into the glass as you wish the liquid to rise. The instant you feel that finger get wet, stop pouring.

Try not to use the glass as a support for the container from which you are pouring, particularly if that container is still full and you are pressing it against the glass as you pour. Holding the glass firmly with your hand in order to use the index finger dipstick will probably avert disaster, but it is better for the hand and forearm of the arm that is pouring to do the work. It is always best to pour fairly quickly, unless you are pouring a carbonated drink.

Let's consider the commonest containers that you pour from now:

Bottles. Place your thumb on the rim of the glass while your finger dipstick is marking a level within the glass, then rest the neck of the bottle lightly on the rim of the glass, bracing it with the end of your thumb as you pour. This allows you to pour with accuracy. It does not hurt to have larger hands if you are using a quart bottle, so men often have an unfair advantage here.

Cans. Smaller cans such as individual servings of fruit juice, soft drinks, and beer, pour easily and present no problems. Large cans are hard to pour from. I am thinking in particular of the large cans of tomato or grapefruit juice that contain forty-eight ounces and are hard for anyone to hold with only one hand. But a large can of fruit juice should not be opened and then placed back in the refrigerator; after as little as twenty-four hours, the juice will taste like rusting can. It is best to pour as much of the can as possible into some kind of storage container, such as a pitcher or large quart jar when you open it. You can safely pour from that second container into your glass.

Cartons. Most milk nowadays comes in paper cartons (smaller than gallon size). Feel along the top ridge of the carton; at one of the ends, you will notice that the ridge is thicker for about three-fourths of an inch. This is the sealed end. Move your hands to the other end, and you will be able to pry open the pour spout with ease. You will generally need both hands to pour from a full-gallon milk carton. The hand that is supporting the side of the carton with the pour spout can also rest on the top of your glass at the same time, and you will not be deprived of your dipstick.

Pitchers, carafes and coffeepots. Easy to pour from, but be careful if you are pouring hot coffee, for example. The dipstick is still just as helpful, but pour more slowly. Your finger will jerk back at the first contact with the hot liquid, which I suppose is a good test of your reflexes. Be sure you have a safe spot to set the hot coffeepot or carafe down on.

I remember the first time I made coffee for friends. After I suggested coffee, one of them stood up and was about to begin the clumsy round of questions: where did I keep the coffee and the coffeemaker, how much to use, where were the cups. I simply got up and did it all myself. It would have been fun to see the looks on their faces, but I could practically feel it. Was I showing off? Sure I was, and it was fun.

One kind of pouring you will want to do almost every day is curiously difficult; pouring boiling water from a small saucepan into a coffee cup or mug. I think working with arcs from two different circles at once is what makes it tricky.

Here is a technique I worked out. You have already put the instant coffee, or tea bag, or cocoa powder, into the cup or mug. Now place the cup or mug as snugly as possible into the front left corner of your sink. This is for right-handed people; if you happen to be left-handed, use the front right-hand corner. Point the handle of the cup or mug straight back towards the back of the sink. Wrap a potholder around the handle of the saucepan. Holding it with both hands, touch the side of the saucepan to the side of the cup until the rim of the pan catches the rim of the cup. Tilt the pan and slide it about two inches up towards the center of the cup. Now raise the pan vertically about three inches, and pour the hot water into the cup.

These may sound like elaborate directions, but they are actually quite simple and become quick and routine. Learn them.

Measuring

Dry measuring. With both dry and wet measuring, you will quickly discover when accuracy is needed and when an approximation suffices. In many of your routine procedures, you will not even need to use special measuring spoons; an ordinary tablespoon can do the job.

It is usually best not to add dry ingredients directly into the cookpot or the mixing bowl. Dry ingredients flow deceptively, and a recalcitrant trickle out of a box or other container may suddenly turn into a small avalanche. Measure first into an extra bowl or saucer, and then remeasure into the larger vessel.

For example, a favorite hot cereal comes, predictably enough, in a box with a pour spout. If too much cereal is dumped directly into the pan of boiling water, it will congeal into a batch of concrete. Better to measure out what you think is the required three tablespoons of dry cereal into your cereal bowl. Then you can spoon the cereal accurately from the bowl into the pan. The extra cereal can then be funneled back into the box.

The same principle applies to seasonings, whether you are preparing food or eating. Don't just shake the salt and pepper over a dish, unless the shaker is a familiar and reliable one. (Obviously it won't be if you are eating at a friend's house or a restaurant.) Instead, shake the salt into the palm of your hand, and then take a pinch of it, just as much as you want.

Naturally, you don't prepare food with dirty hands. If your hands are clean, you can check the level of dry ingredients with your fingers, as you measure them. Also, dipping measuring utensils into spices, herbs, flour and the like presents no problems. But remember to do just that: dip into the dry ingredients. Try not to pour the dry ingredients into the measuring cup or spoon. With spoons the best way to avoid spilling is to use the next larger size. I find it easier to pour a tablespoon one-third or two-thirds full than to fill one teaspoon once or twice neatly and accurately. So use a tablespoon to pour teaspoons and a teaspoon to pour fractions of a teaspoon.

Wet measurings. In general, wet measuring is less tricky than dry. The two liquids that you will be using most are water and milk. It is normal to premeasure them anyway. The real problem is the pouring itself. I use a measuring cup with raised indicators on the outside. I find the proper level indication with my left index finger to match my thumb on the inside of the cup and act as the dipstick. I then pour in the liquid with my right hand, stopping when the liquid touches my left index finger. Often this just means holding the cup under the cold water faucet.

Many of the liquid requirements in these preparations, however, are so approximate that you will find an ordinary measuring cup without any raised markings to be satisfactory. Most dime stores carry plastic measuring cups with raised markings. There is no need to order one from a blind supply house. I recommend that you get one and practice with it.

Timing

I use an ordinary spring-driven kitchen timer that has raised bumps every five minutes on its dial and minute lines in between that I can feel and count with a fingernail. This is not a special gadget for the blind, and can be bought in the housewares section of a department store or a large dime store. You may have trouble timing less than five minutes on this kind of device, if a slight twist of the timer does not supply enough energy to make it tick. So when timing five minutes or less, you may want to set the dial at fifteen minutes and count off the number of minutes you need.

When timing something longer than an hour, such as a roast, I use a braille clock. Many cities have a phone number to call that announces the correct time, and you may choose to use this method too.

The Stove

Skeptics in the audience, both sighted and blind, may be convinced by now that there is much to the notion of coping in the kitchen, without eyes. Where they will draw the line though, and perhaps erect a fence, too, is right in front of the stove: so far and no farther. Admittedly, there is an initial reluctance to the thought of a blind person handling fire, in whatever form. Except for doing without the food itself, though, no other factor would limit food preparation as much as having to go without a stove.

"Playing with fire" is what one friend suggested this section should be called. This is a bad joke because it implies that chance or luck will be more or less responsible for the cook's safety. This is wholly false.

From the standpoint of safety, the most challenging situation is that where the cook is 100 percent blind and intends to use a gas stove. (Antiquated wood and coal burning stoves should not even be considered.) The optimum situation is that where the cook suffers from visual impairment, perhaps legal blindness, and is using an electric stove.

Here are some simple and absolutely inviolable rules for your safety when working at the stove. These rules apply principally to gas flames, but electric stove users should abide by them too.

1. Always be sure where your hands are in relation to the fire. Standing in front of the stove, extend the back of one hand at thigh level and touch the stove. Then make sure you are standing parallel to the stove front, as you move your hands up to the burner controls or to the stovetop.

Turn on a burner. You will hear the sound of the flame coming on. (If you have electronic ignition, you do not have to worry about whether the pilot light is on.) If the flame does not come on, obviously the pilot must be out. You can safely restart the pilot light by lighting the burner itself. Use a wooden kitchen match, not a cardboard match from a match folder. Light the match before turning on the burner. Turn the gas on, very low, and approach the burner cautiously from the front with the lighted match. Presto.

If your pilot lights keep going out, have someone check them to see whether they are getting plugged up and need cleaning.

2. Now that you have turned on a gas burner, it is necessary to adjust it. You must make sure that you know *which* gas cock adjusts *which* burner. And note that the adjustment of the flame is done *without* any cooking vessel resting on the burner.

Hold the flat of your hand about three feet above the burner. Even a hot flame will not hurt you at that distance. Reduce the flame with your other hand, lowering your heat-testing hand *after* you do so, until your test hand is only about a foot or slightly less above the flame. You now have a medium-low flame, appropriate for lots of the food preparations, since I practically always suggest using a low flame. Naturally you can still use a lower flame and will want to with many preparations, but then you will need to be careful that the flame does not go out.

3. If the flame goes out or you want to adjust it higher or lower while cooking, it is always safest to remove the pot or pan to an unlit burner while you adjust the flame.

4. Particularly for women: long, loose or frilly sleeves are obviously messy to cook in, but in addition they are a serious fire hazard. Wear something more practical when you are cooking.

5. Someone had the idea of using a Bunsen burner starter to ignite the burners and the oven of a gas stove without pilot lights. This is one of those bright ideas that does not work. It is dangerous, as I and a friend discovered. Do not try it. To use this hand-operated flint starter safely takes speed, coordination, and above all, eyesight. It presents the double hazard of burning you badly, not just scorching you, and of allowing lots of gas to flow into the air and causing an explosion.

6. There is usually a nice pathway between the two left-hand burners and the two right-hand burners on a stove. Do not place cooking utensils there. When reaching for them while you cook, you run a serious risk of putting your hand too near the flame or touching a hot pan or pot still sitting on a burner. Put all utensils off the stove itself, unless there is a broad area on top of the stove to one side, such as the top of an oven or storage compartment.

7. When you lift a lid from a pan or pot, avoid the temptation of putting it down farther back on the stove. You will probably reach right across the pan or pot in doing this, and risk scalding or burning your forearm. Place lids to one side as you have done with your cooking utensils.

The Oven

Setting temperatures. Stick a piece of plastic marking tape on the stove *front* where the oven dial is turned all the way off. This will usually, though not on all ovens, be at twelve o'clock. Stick another piece of tape on the *dial* where the 350° setting is. When you match the two up, you have a 350°, or a moderate oven, and you will easily be able to judge temperatures above and below this point.

Preheating. It takes about ten minutes to preheat to a temperature of 350°, about fifteen to a hotter oven.

Safety. Always wear a pair of oven mitts when putting anything into the oven or taking anything out. Using only potholders makes it too easy for you to burn the backs of your hands or wrists if they brush against the side of the oven. You not only risk burning your hands, but if that should happen, you may also drop the dish you are trying to put in or take out, spilling the food, breaking the dish, and burning yourself even worse.

When you are ready to remove something from the oven, be sure to turn the oven off first. After you open the oven door, stand back for a full minute while the hottest air rushes out and the oven begins to cool. Then it will be safe and comfortable to put your hands and forearms into the oven.

If a dish is quite heavy or unusually hot, you may wish to set it down on the open oven door while it cools. If you do so, however, you must be sure to remember that you have left it there and that, therefore, the oven door is open. If you do not make a special point of reminding yourself, you will probably walk right into the open door just a few moments later.

Broiler. I advise you not to try to use the broiler. Food such as steaks that you would ordinarily use the broiler for cannot be judged even approximately without eyesight. Cookbooks often state the distance in inches the food should be below the broiler flames, and you cannot judge that either. But to make up for the loss of the broiler, I have included directions for preparing pan-fried steak and pan-fried cheese sandwiches. These are quite satisfactory substitutes for grilling.

Lighting ovens. Judging carefully from my own experience, I advise you not to light the oven yourself if you have to do it by hand with a match. You can still use the oven, but you will have to plan to have someone come by early and light the oven for you. You can put the oven dish in, in advance. I worked out a method for lighting my oven, but it is so tricky and risky that it would be rated Level 4, and I do not even include it here. The only exception I would be willing to make is if you can obtain fireplace matches.

Electric ovens and electronically-ignited gas ovens are thus obviously the best in terms of ease and safety in lighting. Next come gas-piloted gas ovens, which have an annoying tendency to go out. Last come the ovens with no pilot that have to be lighted by hand. I object to this kind, as well as to the oven whose pilot has gone out.

Spreading

Spreading is generally a Level 1 skill, but to spread butter correctly, neatly, and without using your fingers is almost Level 2.

Some spreads are handled best by using a teaspoon alone, without the help of a knife. Examples: egg salad, tuna salad, chicken salad. Dip a heaping spoonful of the spread from its container, place it in the middle of a piece of bread, and spread it around with the bottom of the spoon.

With some other spreads you can choose whether to use only the spoon or use a knife in addition. Examples: jelly, jam, mayonnaise, mustard. Dip a rounded teaspoon of the spread from its container and again deposit it in the middle of a piece of bread. You can now smear it around with the bottom of the spoon if you like; but if you use a knife instead, the spread will be more even and you can cover the corners more neatly. You are allowed to use one finger, of course, to check the corners.

Experience shows that some spreads demand the use of a knife alone, for example, butter and peanut butter.

If you are using butter, make sure that it softens to room temperature. The kind of margarine that comes in a tub usually will be spreadable at refrigerator temperature; stick margarine will not be. With the side, not the edge, of a table knife, feel the end of the stick of butter. Then raise the knife and run the edge about half an inch onto the stick. Cut down. This piece of butter is adequate for a slice of bread. Deposit it in the middle of the slice and spread outwards. I like using stick margarine because tub margarine is harder to measure, and I wind up using my fingers. If you forget to take the butter out of the refrigerator to soften, use a paring knife to cut very thin shavings of butter, and space them on your bread. A hard lump of butter will only dig a hole in the bread if you try to spread it.

Peeling, Slicing, and Chopping Vegetables

These are Level 1 skills, except where onions are concerned. Outwitting this lachrymose vegetable is a Level 2 skill.

The vegetables you will peel most often are cucumbers and carrots. Rinse them thoroughly in cold water before and after peeling. Use an ordinary vegetable peeler; there seems to be only one kind. Always peel away from yourself, using steady, even strokes. It is best to grasp the vegetable at a place behind the point where you start to peel. You can peel about half the vegetable that way, then turn it around, front end aft, and do the other half. Feel with your fingertips to tell whether you have left any unpeeled strips.

Slice the vegetables on a cutting board with a paring knife or serrated steak knife. You will have no difficulty in gauging the thickness you desire.

Onions. First slice off the top and bottom and then peel away the dry outer layer until you expose a fresh, smooth surface. To make fresh onion slices, such as you may like on a hamburger, hold the prepared onion, with your fingers on the lopped-off top and your thumb on the bottom. Press it down firmly on a cutting board. Now slide a knife in underneath your fingers, about three-eighths of an inch from the flat cutoff top of the onion and slice down, firmly and slowly, using sawing motions. Use a serrated knife for this; its teeth will catch so that the knife will not slip and cut your fingers. Repeat this procedure until you have as many slices as you want.

Chopping onions. Prepare the onion as if you were going to slice it. Hold it the same way, but this time cut it straight down through the equator. Now place the hemispheres face down and quarter them. You now have eight chunks, and it is most practical to chop them two at a time in an onion chopper. An onion chopper is one utensil that I find really worthwhile, although in general I am opposed to gadgetry. Any dime store will have one. It is simply a measuring cup whose lid has a spring-loaded plunger with blades at its end passing through it. Do not trust the onion chopper to do a good job without your examining it, though. When you think those chunks are chopped well enough, do not just empty the chopper into the dish you are preparing. Empty the contents first into your hand, and carefully pick through the results. You will often find pieces that need to be put back into the chopper for more work, and also tough pieces of skin that are not crisp enough to use and should be thrown away.

Tears and the onion have engendered all sorts of folk remedies for the problem. Of course, using a closed onion chopper helps. The fine spray of droplets caused by cutting into the onion is responsible for the tears. Somehow they are less potent if you breathe them in through your mouth. And you, as an unsighted cook, have an advantage. Since you cannot watch the onion as you prepare it anyway, close your eyes and turn your head to one side. This is good protection for your eyes, nose, and mouth.

To chop an onion using only a serrated knife, prepare it as if you were going to slice. Now is where technique counts. Place the flat side of the onion half down on a cutting board. Then do *not* grasp it with your left hand and begin carving away with your right; you are as likely to slice the fingers of your left hand as you are the onion. Instead, form an arch with your left hand on top of the onion, slide the knife through it, and cut down. Repeat this procedure several times always using your left hand as an arch over the back of the knife blade; this has the additional advantage of holding the slices of the onion together. Now you need only to rotate the cutting board 90°, repeat the procedure, and you will have chopped the onion half safely and accurately.

What kind of onion to use? The consensus seems to be that yellow onions are better for cooking, white onions are better raw. I particularly like a slice of red Bermuda onion raw on a hamburger.

Steaming Vegetables

This is a way of preparing fresh vegetables that has three advantages over boiling vegetables: it is faster, does not destroy their texture, and saves the vitamins. Boiling vegetables can be slow, tends to make them soggy or mushy, and wastes vitamins, which often are poured down the drain.

The manual skills involved in this operation are peeling or slicing, so it seems to be an easy Level 2 situation. But I am going to label it Level 3 instead, because of the great importance of not steaming you, the cook, as well as the vegetables. By observing one simple safeguard, I have avoided ever being scalded while steaming vegetables. So let me repeat it: when you lift a lid from a pan or pot, avoid the temptation of putting it down farther back on the stove. You will probably reach right across the pan or pot in doing this, and risk scalding or burning your forearm. Place lids to one side.

There are a number of different kinds of steamers, made of metal or ceramic, but there are two general types: the ones that sit on little legs on the bottom of the pan, or those that perch across the top of the pan.

How much better fresh vegetables taste if their texture is slightly firm, crisp, even snappy—depending on the vegetable.

Green beans, carrots, squash, broccoli, and cauliflower are only the most obvious candidates for the process of steaming. Wash and then cut up the vegetables as you want them, remembering that equal size pieces will cook in the same time. Place about three-fourths of an inch of water in the bottom of the pan. Tougher vegetables or ones cut into larger chunks may take more water. The time required is more or less half the time required for boiling, but it is difficult to predict. You will have to test them with a fork for doneness, but do so infrequently. Every time you lift the cover to poke them, the steam escapes and will have to build up again.

When I was a boy, I lived in dread of having certain vegetables appear on my plate—cauliflower, broccoli, brussels sprouts, and asparagus. It wasn't until years later that I realized they had simply been overcooked until they were about the consistency of pablum. With good will, it is possible to spoon down overcooked carrots, peas, or green beans, but transforming those other vegetables into ersatz babyfood is inexcusable. So be sure not to overcook vegetables.

Serving and Eating

Although they are not part of the cooking process proper, serving and eating are part of the continuum that ends only when the dirty dishes land in the sink. Let's not discuss washing them at this point.

Serving. In many American families, particularly those which do not have dining rooms, food is served at the table directly from the cookpot. I strongly recommend against this practice for you, particularly if you are not eating alone. It is simply too hazardous. You serve from the stove to an adjacent workspace or simply move the whole operation to that workspace. If your counter is not heat-proof, place a potholder beneath the pan, then move the dish up to the pan until it touches, and serve.

The relative ease in serving depends largely on your menu; it is more difficult to serve runny dishes such as stews or food prepared in a sauce, or to put gravy on potatoes by yourself. If you are not eating alone, there is no reason not to let someone else do the serving. Your achievement in cooking the meal is striking enough and will be appreciated even more as the meal is eaten. Let someone else dish it up and pass things around.

Eating. Anxiety about being able to eat neatly plagues many blind people. Will I knock over a glass? Scoop food onto the tablecloth or onto the floor? Be stymied when I try to cut the meat? Or put a bare fork into my mouth after I think I've loaded it properly? All of these things can happen and do. Yet they can and should be minimized; the fear of embarrassing oneself and others has spoiled many a meal needlessly. Worse still, inhibitions about eating have caused many a dinner invitation to be declined, thus intensifying the isolation that blind people may suffer from already.

At one extreme of caution, if you are eating alone, you can always rely on the old bowl-and-spoon ploy. If you are eating alone, you will often find it easier to use two or three cereal bowls to eat from, or a bowl and a plate. And since no one is looking, you will be tempted to use a spoon in many instances where you used to use a fork. By all means, take advantage of these solutions occasionally; they are undeniably convenient. But they are also lazy, and if you have come so far as to cook with your handicap, why neglect the finishing touches? I admit that I sometimes eat scrambled eggs from a cereal bowl, but ordinarily it is part of my pride in what I have accomplished to eat as normally as possible.

There are a few simple techniques you can use that are practical and inconspicuous. They will effectively defuse your fear of embarrassment, no matter whether you are eating at home with friends or family, or in the more formal situation of eating out at a restaurant or banquet.

First, go ahead and use your spoon more often than others do. It is particularly useful in eating small bits that you cannot spear, and for cleaning up your plate. You will have plenty of opportunity to ply knife and fork as well. If you have the chance, let your host or hostess know that you would like a serrated knife; they are safer and faster than either an ordinary table knife or a non-serrated steak knife. And you will still have the table knife there to spread butter with.

The clock face. When you tell your friends that your plate is a clock face, they will immediately catch on and even think it's fun: "Your creamed corn is at about two o'clock, the roast is at six, and the potato is at ten. Your salad and a glass of iced tea are crossed together between ten and twelve noon." Without confusion, you will thus be able to choose the right utensil for the job and move it to its place: your spoon for the creamed corn, or knife and fork for the slice of roast, which you can cut for yourself with a little practice.

The locater-backstop. A no-nonsense nurse once told me, "Honey, the others have got two good eyes. It's fair for you to use one finger." Since I am right-handed, the finger I use as a utensil is my left index finger. (Fingers were made before forks, as the saying goes. And who would try to eat fried chicken any other way but with their hands?) That finger comes in most handy: to locate food you have simply forgotten the location of, and help identify it; to mark the individual pieces of meat you have cut, so you can spear them accurately with your fork; and to serve as a backstop when you are worried about pushing food over the edge of the plate. Surprisingly enough, your finger will not get very messy. And you do have a napkin.

Cutting meat. With a serrated knife, and a little practice, you can handle simple slices of meat confidently—roast, steak, ham, liver, and so on. Chops too are quickly mastered, because you know just where the bone is and what it's shaped like. You know approximately where the meat is located on the clock face. With your left hand, slide your fork along until it encounters the edge of the meat. Then place your fork half to three-quarters of an inch in from the edge of the meat—your guess is good enough—and move your knife so that it is parallel to the tines of the fork and touching or almost touching them. Now begin to cut, using slow and firm strokes. The serrations on the knife are particularly good at severing those fibers that you might accidently leave connecting the piece you are cutting from the main piece. The piece you have now cut is the right width; your only other problem is to find out whether it is the right length, as well. If it is too long, reposition your fork and cut the piece in half. Common sense.

Feel free to ask for help. If you think you aren't ready to cut meat yet, or are facing some other problem you cannot or do not want to deal with, just ask whoever's sitting next to you for help. This will seem quite natural to them, and is far better than wrestling (literally) with your food while the others look on with bated breath, or try not to look on. In fact, the problem you are most likely to have is a nice one—politely turning down help that you don't need.

Besides, since you're a guest, you don't have to worry about pouring.

Cleaning Up

Washing dishes. This is a Level 1 skill at best, yet it is the most tedious and unpopular task in the kitchen. I make it a rule not to let dirty dishes pile up from meal to meal. And of all the rules in this book, that is surely the one I violate most often. But do wash dishes after every meal: the fewer there are to clean up, the less tedious it will be.

I happen to disapprove of automatic dishwashers. Even if your kitchen comes equipped with one, you can choose not to use it. Dishwashers are energy hogs—they may use up to sixteen gallons of hot water per load, enough for a leisurely shower. You therefore feel the need to wait until the dishwasher is full to justify using that much hot water, and discover that half of your dishes and utensils are stored, dirty, inside that dishwasher.

Rinse all dirty dishes and place them, gingerly, in a plastic dishpan. Lay all glasses on their sides. Do not put knives into the dishpan; wash them separately. Use water as hot as you can comfortably stand it, both for washing and rinsing. I use a plastic scrubber for everything, except where food has cooked on. As you rinse each dish or utensil, feel it over carefully to make sure you have missed nothing.

I use a metal scrubber for food cooked onto pans and oven dishes. If they are stubborn, let them soak for a few hours. This is the only legitimate excuse for postponing the odious task of dishwashing.

Spilling and breaking. That sounds too much like I'm about to give instructions on how to break and spill. Instead, I'll talk about how not to, and how to clean up after yourself if you do spill or break something.

The possibility of spilling or breaking something, and even more so, the supposed inevitability of cutting or burning yourself, convince many people that blind cookery is unsafe. But the problem of safety, after all, is only a problem of technique. So far, I have never burned myself significantly enough even to raise a blister, and I do not intend to. I admit to having singed a finger more than once, but it has always been due to my sloppy technique. And I have never cut myself. I have, however, slopped, cracked, and smashed on numerous occasions, but never harming myself.

Breaking. I sometimes break things simply by dropping them, but more often I do so by knocking one object against another—most typically, one glass against another. I have simply forgotten that the other glass was there, thereby breaking not only a glass or two but one of the most fundamental rules for proper technique: always remember just exactly where you have put everything.

You should be most careful of all when washing the dishes. Here it is very easy to bump and drop things. Remember that their wetness makes it easy for them to slip out of your hands.

Always remember to use potholders or asbestos mittens to pick up anything hot from the stove or oven. Otherwise you may receive an unpleasant surprise—and drop the hot potato.

Broken glass is a problem. Start by picking up the big pieces but *not* with your bare hands. It is tempting to use them particularly if you are dealing only with a plate or piece of crockery that you sense has suffered a simple fracture. If you do use your bare hands, sooner or later you will cut yourself. Protect your hand in some way. Use oven mitts, a potholder, a towel, something between your hands and the larger pieces of glass. Then use a dustpan and whisk broom or other small hand broom to pick up as many of the smaller pieces and splinters as possible. Because the possibility of stray pieces is so great, be sure to inform the first sighted person who comes on the scene of what has happened and ask him to inspect. Safety first.

Spilling. When you spill a liquid, you have your choice between a sponge and paper towel. I use both. First I mop up the spill with a sponge, and then I use moistened paper towels to wash the floor, followed by dry ones. Use systematic back and forth strokes when you are cleaning, as if painting the floor. Little will escape you. This is nothing but common sense and we cannot even call it a Level 1 skill.

For spilled vegetables or the like, I use a dustpan and sponge. Since vegetables bounce and roll, you will inevitably miss some of them—that's the breaks of the game.

A Note on Electrical Appliances

Americans are in love with kitchen gadgetry, especially electrical appliances. The only electrical appliance you will need for the food preparations in this book is a toaster, but there are three others that will come in handy: a slow-cook pot, an electric coffeemaker, and an electric can opener.

I use an ordinary wall can opener, which is a Level 2 skill. But I'm used to it and have not bothered to buy an electric opener, which is only a Level 1 skill.

I like using an electric coffeemaker, and prefer the type with a drawer to the percolator type, because coffee tastes better if it does not boil. Both kinds are easier to use than a percolator on the stove, because they are self-timing. The best way to load an electric coffeemaker is to pour in, cup by cup, as much water as you want coffee.

The slow-cooker is optional. I like to use it for making chili, spaghetti sauce, and bean and pea soup. The slow-cooking improves the flavor and does not heat up the kitchen in the summertime. There are special cookbooks available for slow-cooking, and you will be able to use these cookbooks without much difficulty.

Who needs to see a toaster to use it? You can adjust the toasting time by touching and smelling the toast. If you are too impatient to wait until the toast cools a bit before you take it out, you can slide a table knife along the top of the toaster until it hits the protruding toast, spear it, and lift it out that way. Be sure you do not stick the knife blade into the toaster.

You will be able to use an electric knife without any problem, although this is another appliance I don't bother with. As a safety measure, be sure you always have a fork in your left hand while you are operating the knife in your right. This will prevent you from using anything but the fork to hold down the meat as you are slicing it.

Operating a food blender is a fairly easy skill, but nothing in this book calls for it. If you have a blender, it almost certainly came provided with recipes for its use.

I recommend that you do not use an electric food mixer. The few times some mixing is called for in this book, a hand-turned mixer is sufficient. Electric mixers simply have too great a risk factor for me to recommend them. They are most useful in baking, and I have given you only a very few, basic baking preparations. Problems of measuring, sifting, and timing make much baking Level 4 preparations, and I have drawn the line at Level 3. If you become skilled enough so that you want to attempt Level 4 preparations on your own, then you must also be skilled enough to face handling the greater potential hazard of the electric mixer.

I have the same recommendation about microwave ovens: do not use them. By federal regulations, most of them are so safeguarded that you cannot hurt yourself by using them. But most of them have a bewildering array of touch panel controls that are rather difficult for a blind person to use. If you have one in your kitchen perhaps someone can tutor you, identifying the control panels with plastic marking tape.

Conclusion

The "Techniques" section ends here. What follows would usually be called the recipe section, but I call it "Food Preparations," in order to stress the importance of techniques versus mere listing of ingredients. If you have understood and mastered the techniques, you have already accomplished a lot. Here is a list of some things you can already do simply by using what you have learned so far. Many other skills and preparations not listed will suggest themselves to you in the natural course of fixing meals and snacks.

You Already Can

In using the techniques in the preceding chapter, you now possess many skills, including some for food preparations without having to refer to Part Two. I have graded the skills Levels 1, 2, or 3, in order of increasing difficulty. Preparations are graded in the same way, according to the combination of skills involved.

Level 1:

Measuring dry materials of all kinds
Pouring cold or warm (but not hot) liquids from cans, bottles, cartons of one quart capacity or less, pitchers and carafes of any size
Opening all cans, jars, bottles, boxes, except for key-opening cans
Spreading various things
Arranging and finding things in cupboards, drawers, refrigerators
Seasoning to taste
Using this book

Level 2:

Pouring from half-gallon or larger containers
Pouring hot liquids, such as boiling water
Measuring liquids accurately for a recipe
Peeling things (a potential safety problem)
Using a spatula
Judging by smell when something in the frying pan is ready
Serving from the stove (also a Level 3 skill)
Using a manual wall can opener

Most of the skills involved in eating at table without resorting to handy "Large Baby" techniques

Level 3:

Using an old-fashioned hand-held can opener

Removing things from the oven (usually very easy, but a potential safety hazard)

Cutting your own pork chop on a plate in a social situation

Eating peas with a fork

Carving a stuffed roast bird

Preparations

Level 1:

Canned or fresh-frozen vegetables

Cold cereals

Toast

Instant cold-drink mixes

Boiling hot dogs

Level 2:

Hot cereals

Dried soup mixes

Canned soups

Most sandwiches

Iced Tea

TV dinners

Packaged hamburger stretchers

Instant potatoes

Fresh-frozen pies

Prepackaged enveloped salad dressings, spaghetti sauces, gravies, sauces, etc.

Powdered milk

Jello

Hot buttered popcorn

Instant coffee

Level 3:

Steaming any vegetable

Part Two

FOOD PREPARATIONS

Introductory Note

I have carefully tested all these preparations myself. Try them my way first, before you make any changes. Again, they are graded Level 1, 2 and 3 in order of increasing difficulty.

Breakfast

Cold Cereal / Level 1

When pouring milk or half-and-half on your cereal, either hold a finger beneath the spout of the milk carton so you can estimate how much is coming out, or hold your finger in the cereal bowl to judge the level of the milk as the bowl fills.

Hot Cereal / Level 2

Don't measure the dry cereal directly into the boiling water; use the remeasuring technique described in Measuring. Be sure to stir the mixture a few times to avoid lumps. Estimate the amount of milk you are pouring into the cooked cereal by holding a finger beneath the spout of the carton only; the cereal is too hot to put your finger into the bowl. A bit of cinnamon makes an attractive topping.

Some hot cereals, such as oatmeal, come in premeasured envelopes of one serving each. You may also find them presugared or flavored in some other way.

Making Toast / Level 1

If you wish to make only one piece of toast, remember that many toasters require you to use one particular slot to do so. Keep that side of the toaster toward you when you set it upon the kitchen counter or table. Toast makes an ideal backstop when you are eating moist scrambled or fried eggs all the time.

Don't neglect the English muffins, popovers, and waffles made nowadays to fit into your toaster; they are convenient breakfast items.

Eggs

Eggs are nature's most versatile food. Whether as an ingredient or as a dish in their own right, any cook uses them everyday. With very little practice, you will be able to prepare eggs for all standard dishes; I am fond of them for the fine and nourishing light supper they can make as well.

Scramble-Fried Eggs / Level 1

This preparation is not just convenient, it is downright lazy. After bacon fat or butter has melted in the skillet over low heat, crack 2 eggs directly into the pan. You need not be careful, since you are about to break the yolks and whites. As the eggs cook, turn them with a spoon so they will cook evenly. When you think they are almost done, scoop up a spoonful and test it with a finger for the degree of moisture that you prefer.

Scrambled or fried eggs should also cook slowly over low heat. Otherwise they will turn too dry or hard before you are aware of it.

Scrambled Eggs / Level 2

Crack 2 eggs into a bowl. (At this point, some cooks like to add a dollop of milk or cream.) Now mix the eggs. Stir them vigorously with a fork, whisk, or hand-turned food mixer if you wish to blend the yolks and whites more smoothly and produce a frothy mixture that is supposed to make the cooked eggs even lighter.

There are many ways to dress up scrambled eggs, ranging all the way from cheese to such exotica as anchovies or caviar. Let's not go overboard, though, and just start with cheese. Cut very small chunks of cheese (American, cheddar, or Swiss does well) into the bowl before mixing. They will melt and blend in adequately. Most of the other popular additives should not be put into the egg bowl but sautéed in the frying pan for a couple of minutes. For example: canned or fresh mushrooms, chopped onions, celery or bell pepper.

If you have not sautéed anything in the frying pan, you will need to add butter or fat at this point. The frying pan—standard 8-inch size is handiest—needs a generous teaspoon of fat: butter, margarine, or bacon grease melted over low heat.

If the egg mixture causes a loud sizzle or even splattering when you pour it in, the heat is too high. Stir 2 or 3 times a minute with a spoon—I like using a wooden spoon, because the handle doesn't heat up. As soon as you feel the eggs thickening, aim less to stir them than to turn them over in clumps so they will all heat evenly. Turn off the heat when you guess the eggs are not quite done. Test them for the moistness you desire while the heat remaining in the skillet cooks them a little more.

Hard-Boiled Eggs / Level 1

Place as many eggs as you want to hard-boil in a saucepan, covering them completely with cold water and then adding another inch. Bring them slowly to a boil and then let them simmer for about twenty minutes. I suggest a relatively long boiling time of 20 minutes because then you will not have to worry about the size of the eggs or their initial temperature. Starting with cold water and bringing them to a simmer slowly help to keep the eggs from cracking as the air in the broad end of the egg heats up.

After boiling, immediately place the eggs in a stream of cold water and let it run over them for about 5 minutes. This will prevent the eggshells from sticking to the eggs when you peel them. Then refrigerate them immediately. (If there is room, place them in the freezer for the first 15 minutes and then transfer them to the main part of the refrigerator.) The reasons for this are aesthetic and practical: the outside of the yolks will not turn green, and the eggshell should peel off cleanly without chunks of the egg white sticking to it.

Soft-Boiled Eggs / Level 2

Place an egg or eggs in boiling water with a tablespoon or serving spoon. Boil for 4 minutes. Lift the eggs out of the boiling water and run under cold water for about 3 to 4 minutes. This stops the eggs from cooking harder in their residual heat and also cools the shell a bit for handling.

Cracking a soft-boiled egg is not an easy job when you can't see it, which makes this preparation a Level 2. I do it this way: fold up a square of paper towel into a belt and place around the middle of the egg. Then, instead of aiming the classic karate chop at the egg with a table knife, I jab into the egg deliberately with a table knife about one third of the way down and saw and pry off the top. Do this over a cereal bowl in which you have already placed a little pat of butter. Now scrape out the egg as best you can. The juggling act with the hot egg is worth it.

Fried Eggs, Sunnyside Up / Level 2

Melt a little butter or fat in a small 6-inch frying pan. Crack 2 eggs into it. If the eggs sizzle loudly or splatter, the heat is too high. Eggs should fry over very low heat.

Deciding when the eggs are done is tricky at first, and sometimes you may wind up with eggs that are too runny or too hard for your taste. Cooking them very slowly gives you more time to judge their doneness, and this will soon become routine. The size of the eggs, how cold they are to begin with, and the exact heat at which they are fried, vary so much that a mechanical timer is of no real help. Shaking the pan gently at intervals will give you a notion of how the eggs are firming up. Also try sniffing cautiously over the pan. A "browning" smell probably means that the whites are overdone. Use a table knife, not a sharp knife, to loosen the edges of the eggs all around the pan. This should give you further evidence of their firmness and whether they need to remain a while longer in the hot pan with the heat off. Then slide the eggs onto a plate using a spatula.

I sometimes use a teaspoon to eat the fried eggs. I like using toast to clean up the plate.

The Unflippable Fried Egg / Level 2

Flipping an egg is not all that difficult, but doing so without breaking it is. Like most fried-egg eaters, I like to reserve the pleasure of stabbing the yolk and spreading it around for the moment when the egg is on my plate and the toast is ready.

Remove the top and bottom from a tuna can; the can is to act as your mold. Put a little more grease than usual in your skillet, and when it has melted, place the tuna can in the center of the pan. Crack an egg carefully on the side of the skillet and then empty it into the ring formed by the tuna can. Cook slowly, basting constantly with spoonfuls of grease scooped up from the edges of the pan. This will fry the top of the egg and turn it white just as if you had flipped it. Now turn off the flame. Slide a spatula under both the egg and its tuna can mold, and lift them onto a plate. Slide the spatula away and using an oven mitt knock the tuna can mold sharply against the plate to dislodge the egg.

Fried Eggs Easy Over / Level 2

I'm one of those finicky egg eaters who prefers his eggs turned over so the whites won't *glitschig,* as the Germans put it.

The technique, though, is a bit tricky at first, and you should be willing to tolerate a few broken yolks when practicing. Fry the eggs as above. You may be able to flip the eggs successfully in the same pan, but I find it difficult. Here is a longer but more accurate way to do it. While the eggs cook, melt butter or fat in a larger skillet. When the butter has melted, turn off the burner. When the eggs are nearly done in the small pan, turn off the burner, loosen the eggs, and turn the pan rapidly upside down over the larger one, and the eggs will flip into it. Count to fifteen, and your eggs are done, easy over.

I find most larger pans too deep to slide the eggs out of without risking further casualties. So, place a dinner plate upside down over the skillet, and, wearing oven mitts, place one hand firmly over the bottom of the plate and turn the pan upside down. Of course, the eggs are now deposited neatly on the plate.

Poached Eggs / Level 2

Bring about 1½ inches of water to a brisk boil in a saucepan. Now turn off the burner, crack an egg on the rim of the pan, and dump the egg into the water. Turn on the burner and poach the egg for 2½ to 3 minutes, not more.

A good way to time the egg is this: toast a piece of bread. Then butter it liberally and place it on a plate. This takes about the length of time that the egg should poach.

Turn off the burner. With a slotted spoon, lift the egg out of the pan and place it on the toast. Because you are using a small pan, the egg will not be able to escape the slotted spoon when you lift it out of the pan.

The Basic Omelette / Level 2

Elegant omelettes require a combination of artistry and sleight of hand. It also helps to be born French. This basic omelette, however, is almost foolproof, and is only one step harder than scrambled eggs.

Crack 3 eggs, not more, into a bowl and add 1 tablespoon of water. Beat with a whisk or a food mixer. Now add any of the ingredients that you might add to scrambled eggs, but chop them more finely. Cheese and mushrooms are the easiest and best. Stir them in with a fork.

Melt 1 tablespoon of butter or margarine in a skillet over medium heat. I prefer a 9-inch nonstick frying pan. When the butter sizzles, turn the heat down to very low. Now pour in the egg mixture. In just a few seconds the eggs will begin to set. Wait 1 minute and then lift one edge of the setting omelette with a spatula. Tip the pan so that the runny eggs on top will flow underneath and set. Do this 2 or 3 times more. The underside should be firm, but not tough or hard; the top should still be quite moist. You can tell when the omelette is finished and is ready to fold by feeling both the underside and the top with the spatula, and by smell. Now, making sure the entire underside is loose, fold the omelette in half with the spatula, like a sandwich, and slide it onto a plate.

The simplest omelette of all can be made by using eggs only, and topping the omelette with a tablespoon of jelly or jam before folding it.

Breakfast Sausage, Links or Patties / Level 1

This meat is extremely fatty, and you should cook off most of the fat, but without overcooking until it's hard.

Links. Fry them over low heat, turning them frequently with a fork to make them cook evenly and keep them from sticking to the pan. They will shrink to about ⅔ of their original size. They are done when you poke them with a fork and they give but still have some resistance. If they break when you poke them, they are overdone. Drain on a paper towel.

Patties. They should be about the size of small hamburgers to begin with, and of even thickness so they will cook all the way through. You can turn them over more easily with a serving spoon than with a spatula. Patties crumble much more readily than links, so try to make the patties as firm and compact as you can when you shape them. Drain on a paper towel.

I do not like to use the leftover sausage grease to fry eggs in. The taste of salt and sage seems to overpower the taste of the eggs. Throw out the grease and start afresh with a bit of butter.

Pan-Fried Bacon / Level 2

I would like to teach you two ways of frying bacon, one way easier than the other.

The easier method I call the hit-or-miss method. Take as much bacon as you want from the package, about 3 strips, perhaps, and cut each strip into 4 pieces. Arrange them in a cold frying pan so they do not touch each other. Then cook them over low heat. When their sizzling diminishes—be patient—that means that most of the available fat has been melted out of the bottom sides. With two forks, turn the bacon over; some of the pieces may stick a little. A random lifting and stirring of the pieces will be the best you can do. You won't be able to identify the pieces individually.

Since the pieces have shrunk, concentrate them more toward the center of the pan, not worrying whether some of the pieces are lying on top of one another. This phase of the frying will go more quickly. Listen again for the sizzling to die down, and also use your nose to make sure the meat doesn't start to overcook or burn.

Remember that pork must not be underdone. Lift the bacon onto paper towels to drain. After about a minute or so, when the pieces are still quite hot, poke them with a fork or a cautious probe with your fingers to tell whether any of the pieces are underdone. If some are, put them back in the pan to fry some more.

The first method gave you a jumble of tasty, rather small pieces. The second requires a little more patience, but has more attractive results. Take only 2 or 3 strips this time, and cut each in half. Now arrange the pieces carefully in a cold pan in a geometric pattern, either 2 rows of 2 or of 3. Fry slowly as before. When they are ready to be turned, you should be able to identify the pieces individually by touch and position as you turn them over using two forks.

The cheapest bacon you can buy at a large supermarket is usually a big 4-pound box of odds and ends. This costs about a third as much per pound as the standard packages, and is a real bargain if you have refrigerator space to store it and the crew to consume it. Of course, these are trimmings and scraps, so they vary greatly in thickness and length. When you have some spare time, sit down with a cutting board and a serrated knife. Sort the pieces according to thickness, and then cut them into 2 or 3-inch lengths. Now pack each pile of like pieces in a plastic bag and put most of it in the freezer compartment; what you have bought will last a long time.

There are various devices on the market designed to eliminate the need to turn over frying bacon at all. Most of them are some sort of perforated sheet of metal that fits down over the cooking bacon. Most of them, I regret to say, also don't work very well. To most bacon lovers, the texture of the bacon—ranging from very crisp to somewhat limp—is almost as important as the flavor, so that is why I have expended so many words on ideas for frying bacon.

Oven-Fried Bacon / Level 1

The more you can simulate the effects of frying within the oven instead of on top of the stove, the less you will splatter and run the risk of burning yourself.

Place strips of bacon on a broiler pan. This is usually a rectangular device consisting of two levels. Bake the bacon on this broiler pan for about 12 minutes in a medium (about 350°) oven. You will not need to turn the bacon over.

Pancakes / Level 2

This may seem like Level 3, but after you do it once, it turns out to be only a Level 2 preparation. Use whatever pancake mix strikes your fancy; it doesn't matter. The one I use combines 1 cup of mix with ¾ cup of water, which makes approximately 6 5-inch pancakes.

Mix the two ingredients in a bowl, using a fork or spoon. No food mixer is necessary. I like to fry the batter in an 8-inch nonsticking frypan, one pancake at a time. That way I can deposit it right in the center of the pan, and know exactly where it is when I want to flip it.

If you use a nonsticking pan, shortening is optional. Otherwise, you need it. Use a scoop large enough so that you can dip out batter for an entire pancake at once. I use a ½ cup flour scoop, not quite full. Let the pan warm up over low to very low heat. Now pour in the batter. Listen closely. As the pancake fries, it will make a soft spluttering sound, not noisy enough to be called a sizzle. As you listen, the spluttering will diminish and slowly come to a stop. When it has almost completely stopped, it is ready to turn. This will take about 3 minutes but go by the sound, not the clock. As an additional test, poke the pancake at this time with a fork. The top should still be runny, and the bottom should give with just about the feeling of a piece of bread. If the temperature is too high, the pancake will begin to smell too brown, and the surface will still be runny while the bottom is too tough.

Move the pan to an unlit burner. Slide a spatula under the pancake and flip it. Since you are only making one at a time, you will not have to worry about getting right underneath the whole pancake or of making it land on top of another one. Now return it to the flame and let it fry for 1 minute more. This time you do want to go by the clock and not by your ears. Place the pancake on a plate and start making another. Stack the ones you complete, and they will stay hot.

Now go ahead and pour your favorite kind of topping on the pancakes. Even friends who know that blind people can cook will not believe that you can make delicious pancakes, not too soggy and not overdone. And it is only a Level 2 preparation.

Rice Pudding / Level 2

This pudding makes a good breakfast as well as a simple dessert. Place 1 cup of already cooked rice (see page 71) in a saucepan. Add 1 cup of milk, 1 tablespoon of butter or margarine, and 2½ tablespoons of sugar. Heat over low heat and stir occasionally until the mixture turns creamy, about 20 minutes. Now stir in ¼ teaspoon of vanilla. Eat hot or refrigerated.

Sprinkle the rice pudding with cinnamon when you serve, and stir in a heaping tablespoon of currants, raisins, or cranberries. Makes 2 servings.

Lunch

Hot Dogs Revisited

In its own way, the humble hot dog is responsible for the writing of this cookbook. My student assistant, Tom Albright, was driving me to Houston for an eye examination. Both of us were in a lousy mood and spoiling for a fight. And after the examination, which had produced no new hope for eyesight, I was feeling very sorry for myself as well. Verbalizing freely to Tom, as I always did, I told him how impossible for me it was to do anything at all in the kitchen. I didn't expect any response from him, and I didn't really want any. I just wanted to sulk. But Tom's short fuse had been ignited: "Do you just want to boil hot dogs for the rest of your life?" he yelled. This snapped me out of my self-inflicted doldrums. On the drive home, I began planning this book.

What my assistant should have told me, of course, was that boiling hot dogs was less than a Level 1 preparation, and I could surely do better than that.

The hot dog is an American institution, and I would no more impugn its place on the American menu than I would ice cream and apple pie. But for the blind, it is the easiest, quickest, and most inexpensive kind of meat to cook, and as such it is in great danger of being overused by us. Yet if it is not overused, the hot dog is a convenient standard that can be enlivened by a couple of easy tasty variations.

Familiarity breeds contempt, the saying goes, but it also engenders contentment. And thus it is with the ubiquitous hot dog. Usually you boil them (indoors) or roast them (outdoors); but variations possible in preparing them range from hot dogs flambé to hot dogs Waldorf. There's no need to get carried away, though; let us just examine a few ways to make the standard wiener a little more interesting.

Hot Dogs and Bacon / Level 2

Slice hot dogs lengthwise, being very careful not to cut through the final hinge of skin. Place bits or a stick of cheese in the hot dog—you may want to add chopped onion or bell pepper too—and then close the hot dog like a sandwich. Wrap a strip of bacon tightly around hot dog in a spiral, skewering it firmly at each end with a wooden toothpick. Fry until the bacon is cooked. You will need to turn the bacon-dog from side to side to do this, but if you turn it upside down, most of the melted cheese will run out.

Pigs in Blankets / Level 2

It wasn't just the name that made me like these when I was a kid. This is a Level 2 hot dog preparation, made convenient by tube biscuits.

Before you begin, set the oven to the temperature indicated on the biscuit tube and let it preheat while you are fixing the hot dogs. The tube of refrigerator biscuits I usually buy contains 8, which is enough for 4 servings. Use a cookie sheet. Press each biscuit flat, making it longer than it is wide. Now spread mustard and pickle relish on each blanket. Place a hot dog the short way across each blanket, and put a piece of cheese on it or next to it. Now wrap the blanket around the pig, pinching it shut at one side. The biscuits are gummy enough to stretch without tearing if you are careful. Do not put the seam side down. If you do, ingredients may leak while baking and stick the cheese and dough to the cookie sheet.

Put the cookie sheet in the oven and let it bake as long as the directions for the biscuits indicate. If you are only making 4 or 6 pigs in blankets, go ahead and cook the rest of the biscuits in the tube as well. They will not keep once the tube is opened.

Sandwiches / Level 1

Few sandwiches are tricky enough to merit the label of a Level 2 preparation. You can make practically any sandwich you desire after covering slicing, chopping, and spreading in the "Techniques" section.

What would we do without sandwiches? Dagwood Bumstead has given his name to the many-layered midnight special. Priscilla's Pop is condemned to helping clean up the leftovers with his cold mashed-potato sandwiches. And the Peanuts gang reward themselves with jelly bread sandwiches fixed by each other, not by Mom.

Here are some commonsensical tips for preparing ham, chicken, egg, or tuna salad sandwiches. All four use at least 1 tablespoon of mayonnaise to bind them together, depending on the desired moisture of the spread. I also use chopped onion in all four.

Ham and chicken salad. Slice the meat into bits with a paring knife; the size of these bits is up to you. 1 cup of cut meat makes 3 ample sandwiches. Add mayonnaise and onion and blend with a fork.

Egg salad. Peel 2 cold hard-boiled eggs, rinse them, and chop into a bowl. The easiest way to do this is simply to hold the egg in one hand and chop it into a bowl with an unsharp table knife. The pieces will fall neatly into the bowl as you cut and you will avoid two problems: how to hold the egg together as you slice, and how to transfer the pieces from the cutting board to the bowl. Add mayonnaise, onion, and a teaspoon of sweet pickle relish. Blend with a fork.

Tuna salad. Take one standard 6½-ounce can of tuna. Drain off the oil and mince in a bowl with a fork. Add mayonnaise and chopped onion. I use a teaspoon of sweet pickle relish in this one too.

Other condiments: chopped celery goes well with chicken salad, mustard with the ham, and dry mustard with egg salad. Fresh parsley goes well with all of them. And you can also add chopped egg to the ham and tuna.

You can dress up a peanut butter sandwich by adding chopped apple, applesauce, or—I'm serious—sliced banana. When I was living in Munich, I missed peanut butter so badly that I scoured the city until I found some peanuts in a health food store. I borrowed a hand-operated meat grinder from the landlady, cranked the peanuts through it, and mixed in butter with a fork. The landlady eyed me suspiciously during the entire operation. Crazy Americans. When she and the landlord tried it, they immediately became converts to the American specialty, and eagerly told the neighbors about this strange *Erdnussbutter* ("earth-nut butter").

Grilled Cheese Sandwich / Level 2

This grilled sandwich is minus the grill, which is too dangerous for you to use safely.

Butter 2 slices of bread liberally. Place 1 slice buttered side down in a frying pan. Cover it with sliced cheese. Place the other piece of bread over the cheese, buttered side up. Cover the pan.

Light a burner and reduce the heat to low. Place the pan over the heat. Heat for 3 or 4 minutes. Cautiously remove the lid and sniff.

Do this every minute or so until you smell the sandwich browning. The sandwich is now ready to be turned. Be careful—this is harder than you think.

Turn off the heat. Slide a spatula underneath the sandwich, making sure that it is exactly and fully beneath the sandwich. If you cannot tell this by the heft of it, simply touch it all around with a fork. Lift the sandwich slightly, making sure that no melted cheese around the edges has glued it to the pan. Use the fork to free it if it is stuck. Now lift the sandwich up about 6 inches more and flip it. Do not do so too vigorously, or you will throw it and it may slide apart. The second time you perform this operation, it will seem perfectly natural to you and will require no thought. Again, cover the pan. The second side will brown much faster than the first. When it is done, slide it onto a plate with the spatula. It will be very hot. Cut it in half and let cool for a couple of minutes.

Reuben Sandwich / Level 2

This sandwich gets its name from Arnold Reuben, the American restauranteur who first created it.

Sauerkraut seems like a strange sandwich ingredient, but it gives the combination of Swiss cheese and corned beef its authority. Butter 2 slices of rye bread, whatever variety you like. In layers, put down a slice of canned corned beef, some sauerkraut, and a slice of Swiss cheese. Spread French or Russian salad dressing on the cheese. Wrap the sandwich in aluminum foil and bake at 350° for about 25 minutes. When you take the sandwich from the oven, place it on a plate while unwrapping it.

Hamburgers / Level 2

I'm not trying to cover the field, only to show you the way I usually make hamburgers. Most fast food chains charge a dollar or more for a hamburger so it is a good idea to be able to make them at home.

I usually buy 1 pound of ground beef at a time and divide it into 4, because a ¼ pound of meat makes an ideal burger. I wrap 3 chunks individually and store them in the freezer.

First decide whether to mix anything into the raw beef. Chopped onion, dried onion flakes, or parsley are possibilities. Then shape the meat into a patty with your hands. Do not just press it flat with a spatula, because you cannot be sure then if it will hold together. Place it in the center of a skillet. If the skillet is not stick-proof and you are using lean ground beef instead of regular, put a pat of butter underneath the burger.

You want to cook the burger 5 minutes on each side over medium-low heat. Turn on the heat, set your timer for 10 minutes, and shake a little salt and pepper on the burger. I like flavoring it with a couple dashes of Worcestershire sauce at this point. You can try steak sauce if you like. When 5 minutes are up, turn the burger with a spatula and add a little salt, pepper, and sauce to the other side.

Now is time to add the slice of cheese if you are making a cheeseburger. You will need to cover the pan so that the cheese will melt.

Macaroni Salad / Level 2

This lazy preparation should please everyone. Try it the next time you are asked to contribute a dish to a picnic or a summer potluck supper. The proportions given here provide enough for about 4 ample servings.

Dump about a cup of macaroni elbows into a large saucepan of boiling water. Stir occasionally so that the macaroni will not stick to itself or to the pan. If you have a timer, set it for about 12 minutes. But it is easy to judge roughly 10 minutes, and then begin testing the macaroni to see if it is done by sticking a table fork into the boiling water to see if you come up with some macaroni on it. Give it a few seconds to cool, and then chew it to see whether it is cooked soft enough.

If it is done, dump the saucepan into a sieve in the sink and run cold water over the macaroni, rinsing it thoroughly. Place it in a covered bowl in the refrigerator overnight.

Before you are ready for your outing the next day, prepare egg salad as described on page 64. Mix it in well with the cold, cooked macaroni. Tomato slices make a juicy addition.

Dishes like macaroni, tuna, or chicken salad are often responsible for food poisoning at picnics, since they spoil so quickly in the hot sun. Keep the salad covered and in an ice chest until it is time to serve it. And if you are eating both early and late, cover the salad and put it back in the ice chest.

Hearty Bean Soup / Level 2

I tried out various bean soup preparations, but finally settled on this one, which I improvised one chilly winter afternoon.

Put a ½ pound of small white beans in a quart jar, fill the jar with water, and let the beans soak overnight. They will swell up to fill most of the jar.

Pour the beans and water into a slow-cook pot, and add the following ingredients: 1½ pints more of water, ½ teaspoon of salt, 1 bay leaf, 1 teaspoon oregano, ⅓ teaspoon of chopped yellow onion, and the secret ingredient: 3 ounces of molasses.

Now comes the meat. I sliced up 3 wieners, because they were cheap and handy. But almost any kind of cooked pork or beef will do. It's a good way to use up leftovers. Now let the soup simmer in the slow-cooker for at least 12 hours. Serves 6.

Split Pea Soup / Level 2

Empty a 1-pound bag of split peas into a quart jar. Fill the jar with cold water and let it stand overnight. By morning the peas will have absorbed the water and swollen almost to fill the jar. Dump the peas into a kettle or 3-quart pan. Add 1-quart water, 1 bay leaf, 1 teaspoon of salt, ½ teaspoon of pepper, and at least ½ teaspoon of chopped onion. If you have a hambone, put it in too. Bring to a simmer, cover, and let simmer for an hour. Check the water level periodically, and add more water if needed. Stir to keep the peas from caking together. After an hour, add some meat, preferably pork. Chopped up leftover ham is ideal, but in a squeeze, I have even sliced in 3 or 4 hot dogs. Smoked ham hocks, recommended in so many pea soup recipes, are a sham and a disappointment. After 2 or 3 hours of simmering, they remain hard as rock and impossible to eat.

Chopped celery and carrots are often added to traditional pea soup. Try chopping in 1 big celery stalk including the leaves, and 2 medium-sized carrots. You may also want to add garlic or garlic salt, then simmer for an hour more. If you like slow cookery, you can prepare the soup in a slow cookpot for several hours.

Chicken Soup / Level 2

There is nothing wrong with canned chicken soups. But if you have roasted a chicken following the preparation on page 91, and also made chicken pie out of most of the leftovers, let's use it up right down to the last bone.

Take the carcass and put it into a kettle, covering it with water. Bring to a boil and add some chopped onion, celery, carrots, and parsley. Cover the kettle and let it simmer for 2 hours. All those little bits of meat that are hard to get at, such as on the back, will be utilized in this way. Strain the mixture through a sieve to remove the bones and the vegetables. The leftover liquid is called chicken stock, and you can make chicken soups from it effortlessly by merely adding noodles, barley, or rice. Salt to taste.

Devilled Eggs / Level 3

I call this a Level 3 preparation simply because you need to be careful and patient in cutting the eggs and removing their yolks. People are sure to compliment you, because this snack seems to take ingenuity and skill.

Start with 6 hard-boiled eggs (See p. 53). Peel them very carefully and rinse them. Cut the eggs in half lengthwise, and carefully poke or pry the egg yolk out with tip of paring knife, letting it drop into a mixing bowl. Place the egg whites face up on a plate, forming a circle.

In a smaller bowl mix the following ingredients: 1 tablespoon each of mayonnaise, french dressing, soft butter and sour cream (you may substitute another tablespoon of mayonnaise if you do not have the sour cream), ½ tablespoon of vinegar, 1 teaspoon of sugar, ½ teaspoon of powdered mustard.

Blend these well with a fork. Now crumble the egg yolks with the fork, making sure not to pack the yolks together. Add the mixed ingredients and stir. Fill the egg white casings, a heaping teaspoon at a time, going around the circle. Sprinkle the top with paprika.

Many variations may occur to you. I have tried sweet pickle relish, devilled ham spread, and caviar with good results.

Vegetables

Rice / Level 1

Need I argue the economy and ease of cooking with rice? It will be one of the most often employed and versatile of your kitchen repertory. Most rice cooks agree on the following guidelines: always make sure that the water is boiling briskly before you add the rice. Keep the liquid boiling actively while the rice is cooking, because this prevents sogginess. If you need to add more liquid to boiling rice, the additional liquid too should be boiling. Don't stir rice with a spoon, which mashes the grains and makes them gummy; use a fork. Refrain from checking often if you are cooking rice with an exactly measured amount of liquid in a covered pot; it lets steam escape and lowers the temperature. Sometimes, however, you have to check if you think that more liquid needs to be added.

Rice can be kept in the refrigerator, covered, for about a week. Rice can be frozen for about six to eight months. To reheat, place just enough liquid in the bottom of the pan to steam the rice and prevent it from scorching.

A rule of thumb: 1 cup of uncooked white rice plus 2 cups of liquid yield 3 cups of cooked rice; 1 cup of brown rice plus 2½ cups of liquid yield 4 cups of cooked rice.

Coleslaw / Level 1

Why does coleslaw cost so much at the grocery store or delicatessen, when it's made out of something so cheap as cabbage? And it's only a Level 1 preparation! Call it Level 1½ if you get bored doing all that chopping.

Use a large cutting board for your base of operations, because bits of cabbage will be flying about. Slice off about ⅓ of an average-sized cabbage. Discard the outer withered leaves and cut the cabbage into chunks. Now chop them up, a chunk or two at a time, in an onion chopper. Cabbage chops more easily and quickly than onions, but wear an oven mitt to protect your hand from a possible blister because the chopping process takes about 15 minutes.

Empty the chopped cabbage into a large mixing bowl, larger than you think you will need. Add ½ a bell pepper, chopped, and stir in 3 tablespoons of mayonnaise with a fork. In a cup, mix together 2 teaspoons each of sugar and vinegar and 1 teaspoon of concentrated lemon juice. Since accuracy is not important and it is difficult to pour a level teaspoon of liquid, use a tablespoon and guess when you have poured into it ⅔ vinegar or ⅓ lemon juice. Pour this solution over the cabbage and toss again with a fork. This will yield about 3 cups of slaw. Cool it in the refrigerator for about 2 hours before serving to give the slaw a chance to steep in the sweet-sour solution.

Salad Dressing / Level 1

There are many excellent commercial salad dressings available, but the high price charged for such small amounts has always bothered me. Particularly if you like a seasoned vinegar and oil dressing, you should do it yourself.

In a pint jar, combine 8 ounces of olive oil, 4 ounces of red wine vinegar and 3 ounces of water. You can use ordinary salad oil and ordinary vinegar if you want, but these are better. Add: 1 teaspoon of seasoning salt, ½ teaspoon parmesan cheese, ⅛ teaspoon or one pinch each of some kind of Italian seasoning, dried onion flakes, garlic salt, dried mustard, and ¼ teaspoon of black pepper. Shake like mad.

Bean Salad / Level 2

This Level 2 preparation leaves you with lots of halves left over, so go ahead and double it if 8 helpings of bean salad is not too much for you.

In a mixing bowl put half of a 16-ounce can of green beans, and half a can each of wax and kidney beans. You can substitute garbanzo beans, if you like. Cut a white onion in half at its equator. Peel one half, slice it, and pull the slices apart into rings. Add them to the beans. Cut half a bell pepper into thin slices and add them too.

Measure ¼ cup vinegar and ¼ cup salad oil into a jar. Cover the jar and shake it vigorously. Pour the contents over the bean salad and mix the ingredients with a fork. Put the salad in the refrigerator for at least an hour before serving.

Acorn Squash / Level 2

There are three different ways to prepare this winter squash, and they apply to other winter squashes as well, such as butternut, buttercup, banana, and hubbard squash.

For acorn squash: rinse, dry, and cut them in half. Scrape out the seeds with a spoon. Now rub them inside and out with vegetable oil. You may use butter instead, and salt lightly. Place them right side up in a baking pan and bake in a 375° oven for 45 minutes or until fork tender in the middle.

Two slightly different methods: place some water in a pan below the baking pan on a different shelf of the oven to produce steam. Or place the squash with the cut side down in the pan, adding a little water directly to that pan. This will make the squash softer. It is up to you to gauge the difference in taste. Be sure to serve the squash with plenty of butter.

Baked Summer Squash with Cheese / Level 2

Start with 3 medium-sized crookneck yellow squash, or about enough to make 3 cups when sliced. You can also use other summer squash such as patty pan or vegetable marrow. Wash and slice them in ½-inch thick slices. Chop up half of a yellow onion and grate a cup of cheddar cheese. You will also need bread crumbs.

Boil or steam the squash for about 5 minutes. Drain. Now oil a baking dish. Arrange the ingredients in four layers: the squash at the bottom, then the onion, then the cheese, and finally the bread crumbs on top. Bake in a 350° oven for 45 minutes.

An Italian variation uses zucchini, with the addition of 1 can of sliced tomatoes. Drain the can of tomatoes, saving the juice. (The next time you are fixing tomato soup, add this tomato juice instead of the amount of water directed on the soup can.) Prepare the baking dish as before, adding the tomato to the onion layer, along with a ¼ teaspoon of an Italian herb such as oregano.

Creamed Onions / Level 2

These small onions, called boiling onions, usually come in a string bag at the grocery store. Take 10 or 12 of them and peel off the dry skin with your fingers. No other preparation is needed at this point. Boil them until tender. Drain and let them cool until you can handle them. Now you can slice off the tip and base much more easily than you could have when they were raw.

For the sauce, melt 2 tablespoons of butter in a saucepan over low heat. Or if you have a tub of soft margarine, you can spoon it right out. Now add 1 tablespoon of flour, and stir the butter and flour together slowly with a spoon. Then stir in 1 cup of milk: the best way to do this is to add the milk splash by splash. Set down your measuring cup between splashes so you can hold on to the pan with one hand and stir with the other. Now stir in another tablespoon of flour until the mixture comes to a barely audible simmer. The sauce will start to thicken rather rapidly, just about when you think it is not going to thicken at all—in about 5 minutes. You can tell if the sauce is as thick as you like it by dripping it from your spoon. Pour the sauce over the onions.

Guacamole / Level 2

The avocado is ripe enough for guacamole if it gives slightly when you squeeze it with your fingertips. Slice the avocado in two lengthwise around its pit. If the avocado is ripe, you can pry it apart easily with your fingers or a table knife. Remove the pit from one of the halves. Instead of trying to peel off the skin of the avocado, scoop out the meat with a spoon. If you do this gently, the tough skin will not break. Spoon into a bowl and mash with a fork.

Now add these ingredients: 1 chopped tomato and 1 chopped scallion; you can chop these two at the same time in an onion chopper. Then add ½ teaspoon each of chili powder, olive oil, lemon juice and salt, and 1 dash of pepper. These ingredients are optional: ¼ teaspoon coriander, a pinch of cumin powder, and a dash of tabasco sauce. Stir together with a fork. This is a good party dip, or you can serve it as salad on lettuce.

Baked Potatoes / Level 1

The classic Idaho or the Burbank potatoes are best. Scrub them with a plastic or metal scrubber. Feel them over carefully, and with the tip of a paring knife remove any blemishes or eyes that are beginning to sprout.

Rub the potatoes lightly with oil to prevent the skins from hardening. Puncture them a couple of times with a fork and bake them for 45 to 60 minutes in a 450° oven, depending on their size.

Put on your oven mittens. Open the oven and pull the rack way out when you think they are done. Hold a potato down with one hand and puncture it with a serving fork with the other. If the potato gives in smoothly to the fork and there is no hard center, it is done.

Enhance the potato as you please, with salt and pepper, butter, sour cream, grated cheddar cheese, chopped chives, or bacon bits. When you have finished digging out the potato, cut its jacket in half, butter the insides, fold them shut and eat it with your fingers. The skin tastes great and contains many vitamins.

American Fries / Level 2

I won't specify amounts here. Scrub and pare your potatoes. Slice thinly and evenly. Add enough cooking oil to a frying pan to cover the bottom of the pan liberally. Your fingertip will tell you what "liberally" means. Fry the potato slices over low heat, turning often with a spatula. You will smell them browning, and a fork will tell you when the outside surface is turning crusty while the inside is still soft—about 10 minutes.

You can fry thin onion slices at the same time if you wish. You can add salt, pepper, and catsup on your dinner plate.

German Fried Potatoes / Level 2

This is a good way to use leftover boiled potatoes. Cut the potatoes into bite-sized slices; they do not have to be even or of the same size. Pour a thin layer of oil into a skillet, or use bacon drippings. Fry the potatoes over medium heat for 10 minutes or less, stirring and turning so that they do not stick. Salt and pepper to taste. Many people like catsup with any kind of fried potatoes.

Hash Brown Potatoes / Level 2

This is a favorite side dish for a hearty breakfast. Proceed as with the German fries, only cut the potatoes up into smaller pieces, practically crumbled. Use more oil or fat. Cook over medium high heat, at first turning with a spatula and then pressing the mass of the potatoes down so that they will brown and turn crisp.

Scalloped Potatoes / Level 2

Butter the bottom and sides of a 2-quart casserole. Slice thinly about 6 raw potatoes, medium in size. Russets or an all-purpose potato such as a New York potato are recommended. New potatoes are not. Put down a layer about three slices thick in the casserole. Sprinkle the layer with a scant tablespoon of flour, and dot with a teaspoon of butter. Add salt and pepper. Scatter in chopped cheese and/or ham. Continue the layering process until the potato slices are used up. Do not sprinkle anything on the top layer. Now pour in milk until all the cracks are filled and the milk reaches the top of the potatoes. This may take as much as a quart of milk. The milk tends to bubble up, so leave at least an inch at the top of the dish. Now bake in a low oven, 300° for 3 hours. If your casserole dish is not deep, the potatoes may be done in only 1½ to 2 hours. Serves 6 to 8.

Cold Potato Salad / Level 2

You can make potato salad from whatever potatoes you have on hand, although new potatoes are especially nice. For 4 servings, boil enough potatoes to amount to 2 cups, by your guess, or cut-up potatoes afterwards. It is the usual practice to peel the potatoes when they are still warm, but if you have cleaned and pared them properly, there is no need to peel them at all. The peel adds taste, texture and vitamins.

If you would like to marinate the potatoes, try using the salad dressing given on p. 72 for the marinade. Pour half a cup over the potatoes and let it stand for half an hour. Now chop and add those characteristic potato salad ingredients that everyone knows: hard-boiled eggs, celery, pickles, olives, scallions, radishes, cucumber. Stir in mayonnaise and refrigerate. If you did not marinate, you will need to add salt, pepper, and mustard.

German Style Potato Salad / Level 2

Scrub 6 potatoes and pare out any blemished spots or budding potato eyes. Boil them for 35 to 40 minutes, or until very tender. Use medium or medium-small potatoes, or a dozen very small new potatoes. Since it is hard to judge the potatoes' sizes, you will have to test the tenderness of the boiling potatoes every 5 minutes. Let the texture of the potatoes be the judge of when they are ready, not the clock.

While the potatoes are cooking, fry 6 slices of bacon until crisp. Drain the potatoes, replace them in their pot, and crumble in the bacon. Add ¼ cup of bacon drippings, 1 chopped hard-boiled egg, and 1 tablespoon pickle relish. Crush the potatoes with a fork or potato masher. In a measuring cup, combine ¼ cup vinegar, 1 tablespoon sugar, 1 teaspoon onion flakes, ½ teaspoon of paprika. Stir this mixture into the potatoes. If you have done things in this sequence, the potatoes will still be quite hot enough to serve. You can reheat them as leftovers in the oven.

Onion Cheese Potato Cakes / Level 3

This solid peasant fare is a not so distant relative of the German *Kartoffelpuffer,* or potato pancake. The uncooked mixture will not keep, so fry up all the cakes you have supplies for. The fried cakes keep well in the refrigerator and taste as good as fresh when warmed up.

In a mixing bowl combine: 1 medium large russet (Idaho) potato, grated; ½ an onion, chopped; and about 3 ounces of grated cheddar cheese. Scrub the potato well first and pare out any eyes or bad spots, but do not peel it. Crack in 1 egg and add about 3 heaping tablespoons of flour to act as a binder. Stir well with a fork.

Pour cooking oil into a skillet to a depth of about ¼ inch. When the oil begins to sizzle, carefully put in cakes that you have molded with your hands. You can do this by placing each hand-formed cake on a spatula and slipping it into the oil; this way you will not splash any hot oil on your hands. Cover and fry over a medium-low flame for about 8 to 10 minutes. Then turn the cake with a spatula, cover again, and fry for an additional 5 minutes. If you suspect that you are cooking the cakes too rapidly, your nose can detect the smell of the edges beginning to scorch and you can reduce the flame. Salt and pepper to taste. The potato cakes taste delicious with a side dish of applesauce or almost any canned or fresh fruit. Also try them with honey. Yields 4 to 6 cakes.

This recipe sounds foolproof, but it is not quite. If the batter is cooked too hot, the cheese may melt right out of the cakes and stick to the bottom of the pan. This not only eliminates the tastiest ingredient; it also leaves you with a frying pan that is very difficult to clean. If you have a frying pan made of some nonstick material, use it. You will also need less cooking oil in the nonstick pan.

Dinner

Cheese and Meat Casseroles / Level 2

These are among the simplest full-meal dishes.

They can be varied almost endlessly, depending on what leftovers you find in your refrigerator. They are wholesome, filling, and inexpensive. And of course they taste good, or I wouldn't have included them. They are what I use to call "bachelor cooking," because you can make up a lot of it and count on it to last for several meals. I'll describe the ground rules and let you take it from there.

You need three ingredients: carbohydrates in some form, protein, and something that will bind them.

For instance:

Carbohydrate. Use elbow or shell macaroni, flat noodles, or rice. Which carbohydrate goes best with what protein is rather arbitrary, but most people prefer cheese—macaroni with cheese, for instance. Rice with chicken is another combination.

Protein. These dishes are a good way to use up leftovers—beef roasts of any kind, ham, pork roasts, veal, lamb, chicken or turkey. Ground beef and tuna can be stretched in this way, more cheaply by far and tastier than by using the stretcher kits available at the grocery store.

A binder. Use a half a cup of milk, with some powdered milk added as you wish, or a can of some kind of creamed soup, undiluted. I prefer cream of mushroom, but cream of celery and cream of chicken are good too. Use mayonnaise only in cold combinations like the tuna and egg described below.

First prepare the carbohydrate. I suggest 1½ cups, before cooking, of macaroni or noodles, but only 1 cup of rice, which expands more. This corresponds to about 1½ cups of grated cheddar, Swiss or American cheese, or of chopped meat.

Examples:

Macaroni and cheese. Cook the macaroni. While it is boiling, grate the cheese right into an oven bowl. Pour in a ½ cup of milk and up to a ½ cup of dried milk (optional). Stir thoroughly with a fork. Drain the macaroni through a sieve or colander, add it to the bowl and stir. Grate some more cheese over the top. Heat in a 350° oven for 25 minutes.

You can add a cup or more of chopped meat to this to make it even more substantial. I like ham the best with cheese.

Meat casserole. Prepare your carbohydrate. Place it in an oven-proof dish and add about a cup and a half of any kind of chopped leftover meat, or as much previously browned ground beef. Add a can of cream of mushroom or celery soup and stir well. Heat for 20 minutes in a 350° oven.

With leftover chicken, I prefer rice and a can of cream of chicken soup.

There are various ways to add vegetables to these hot casseroles, but by far the simplest is to add one can of peas, drained, to any of the above. Corn or chopped onion are other examples. And of course you have an open invitation to add any herbs you wish. Dried parsley or fresh parsley are good ones. Salt and pepper to taste.

Cold tuna and egg salad. Prepare the macaroni the night before and refrigerate. Combine it in a mixing bowl with 1 can (6½ ounces is standard) of tuna, drained; 2 chopped hard-boiled eggs; 2 heaping tablespoons of mayonnaise; and 1 tablespoon of sweet pickle relish. Stir well. You may add chopped onion or some mustard, either wet or dry, if you want to sharpen the taste. You can substitute cold ham for the tuna, but cold roast beef does not seem as attractive. I like to take a refrigerator dish of this cold salad to work for my lunch. It is a welcome relief to the eternal lunchtime sandwich.

Zucchini Casserole / Level 2

Start with 3 zucchinis about 6 inches long and an inch in diameter, or 1 package of frozen sliced zucchini. Cut them into 1-inch long pieces and put them into a 1-quart buttered casserole dish. Chop up half a green bell pepper, and half an onion, sauté them and add to the zucchini. Then add one 8-ounce can of tomato sauce. Now top with bread crumbs, adding a few dabs of butter to the crumbs here and there. Cook in a 350° oven for 30 minutes, or until the zucchini is fork-tender.

Meat Loaf / Level 2

The meat loaf is about as American as the hamburger, and not that distant a relative of it. Any meat loaf is a reliable Level 2, although there are countless variations.

Mix these ingredients thoroughly in a big bowl with your hands: 1 to 1½ pounds of ground beef; 1 slice of bread, dampened in water and torn into little pieces; 1 finely chopped yellow onion; 1 egg, beaten; ¼ teaspoon salt.

Bake in a loaf pan at 350° for 1 hour.

Meatloaf Variants:

Flavor with catsup, mustard, or Worcestershire sauce.

Use about a ½ cup of cracker crumbs instead of a piece of bread.

Top the loaf with 1 can of cream of mushroom soup, undiluted.

Bake 1 hour, covered with aluminum foil, then uncover and bake for 15 minutes more.

Start with 1 pound of ground beef and ½ pound of ground pork.

Use ¼ cup of rolled oats, ½ cup of milk and ¼ cup catsup.

Substitute 1 envelope of dried-onion soup mix in place of the onion. Add 3 tablespoons of water.

Fried Eggs on Canned Meat / Level 2

Cut 2 slices of any of the precooked meat that still comes in the can with a key opener—Spam, Treet, or the like. Fry them over a low flame (you may use a little butter) until they are piping hot and have begun to turn crisp; turn by using a fork or a spatula. Now set them aside on a plate.

Move the frying pan to a burner that is off, add some more butter, and crack 1 or 2 eggs into it. (You will worry much less about burning your fingers if the pan is not sitting on the heat.) Return the pan to the original burner, which is still on, fry the eggs to the desired consistency, and then slide them onto the meat.

This is a tasty, quick supper, and can be eaten neatly by using a piece of bread or toast as a pusher and mop. It is the equivalent of the German *Leberkäs,* a favorite at many German lunch counters. The only tricky part of this food preparation is opening the can; many can openers will not do the job, and the key is dangerous. If you can, ask someone else to do so for you in advance and put the meat in the refrigerator. After all, it is specially prepared not to spoil.

Tamale Pie / Level 3

I have probably had a dozen different versions of tamale pie. I developed this Level 3 variation myself, and I think you'll like it.

It's a good company dish and has nothing controversially hot about it.

Brown 1 pound of ground beef in a large, heavy skillet and drain the grease if there is any. Now add the following to make the body of the pie: one 16-ounce can of tomatoes, cut up, with juice; 1 small can of corn, drained; 1 4-ounce jar of pimentos, chopped (optional); 1 bell pepper and 1 yellow onion, chopped; 1 can pitted black olives, drained whole. And this for seasoning: ½ teaspoon oregano, ¼ teaspoon each of cumin seed and black pepper, 1 teaspoon garlic salt, and 1 tablespoon chili powder. Simmer for 15 or 20 minutes, depending on how moist you think the pie should be.

While the contents of the pie are simmering, make the topping without which the pie would not be a pie. Pour ¼ cup of cold water into a bowl and stir in 1 cup of corn meal, preferably yellow, bit by bit. Now bring 2 cups of water to a boil and add the corn meal mush and stir it. Cook until it becomes pasty. You can judge the texture by letting the mush drop from a fork or spoon.

Pour the pie contents into a deep oven dish, and spread the topping over it with a large spoon. Add several pats of butter to the topping. Cook in a 375° oven, uncovered, for about 30 minutes, until the topping begins to turn crusty in spots. Test it for crustiness with a fork.

Easy Enchiladas / Level 3

Mexican food is so good that you should have a couple of the basic recipes at your command. Nowadays, most supermarkets even in the North have a small Mexican food section where you can find the tortillas and enchilada sauce called-for here.

Let's make a dozen cheese enchiladas: in a large bowl, mix ¾ pound of cheddar cheese, grated; 1½ onions, chopped; and 5 or so pitted black olives, halved. Put 2 cans of enchilada sauce in another bowl. Now grease a shallow baking pan.

Using tongs, warm each tortilla in hot oil for about 30 seconds, until pliable. Lift and place in the enchilada sauce. This will cool the tortilla so that you can fill it with your hands, roll it shut, and place it seam side down in the baking pan. Pour the remaining sauce over the dozen enchiladas and bake in a 350° oven for 35 to 40 minutes.

You can make chicken enchiladas by cutting the cheese in half and adding as much chopped leftover chicken as you like, with or without the olives. Or to make beef enchiladas, simply brown a pound of ground beef and stuff only with beef and onions.

Chili for Yankees / Level 2

This is a tame and Americanized version of the real thing, that everyone can enjoy without feeling like an active volcano. The real stuff is called "Texas Jailhouse Chili" and originated in the tough but poor hoosegows along the Mexican border. The ingredients were the cheapest that could fill the prisoners' bellies—pinto beans; rattlesnake, rat, and whatever roaches were unlucky enough to fall into the kettle (no ground beef, of course); plus enough ground and dried chili peppers to anneal the taste of anything.

This is a basic and simplified preparation which you may experiment with to your heartburn's content.

Brown 1 pound of ground beef in a large, deep skillet. Spoon off and discard all fat. Add: 1 finely chopped white or yellow onion, 1 15-ounce can of tomato sauce, 2 15-ounce cans of red kidney beans, 1 tablespoon of chili powder, and ½ teaspoon of garlic salt. For more moisture, you may wish to add sliced tomatoes, fresh or canned. (Optional but suggested: 1 bay leaf, ¼ teaspoon of cumin seed.) Cover, stir occasionally, and let simmer for at least 1 hour.

Your results will be even better after browning the ground beef, if you complete the cooking process in an electric slow-cook pot. Also, you cannot really make too much chili, it freezes very well.

Store it in individual, meal-sized containers in your freezer and you'll always have a quick, trouble-free supper on hand.

It is even cheaper to begin with uncooked kidney beans. Empty a 1-pound bag of kidney beans into a sieve. Feel the beans with your fingers and discard any that feel rough or spoiled. Rinse the beans and put them into a large pan or kettle. Cover with 2 inches of water and bring to a fast, audible boil. Turn off the heat and let them stand for an hour. Then bring to a boiling point and let the beans simmer for 1 to 1½ hours, until they are soft.

You can also add chopped bell pepper or pimentos to the chili without making it hotter. It is the fresh or pickled peppers, usually jalapenos, that add the real heat to chili and have given it a diabolical reputation among the innocent. Try putting a couple of chopped jalapenos on the table in a side dish for braver souls to experiment with. It may double their consumption of beer, which remains the ideal beverage with a chili supper.

Beef Stew, Marinated / Level 3

The least expensive cuts of beef include chuck, rump, and round steak. Left untreated, they are often tough. For a little more money per pound, your meat department debones, trims the fat, slices these cuts into chunks and labels them simply "stew meat." Place 1 to 1½ pounds of stew meat in chunks in 1 cup of cheap red wine in a bowl in your refrigerator, for at least 12 hours, preferably 24.

Melt 3 tablespoons of shortening in a heavy skillet or Dutch oven. Spoon the beef chunks into this pan and pour the marinade into a cereal bowl. Brown the chunks of beef over medium-low heat for about 5 minutes, turning them to brown on all sides.

Now set the beef aside; it would be convenient to put it back in the empty marinade bowl. Now sauté 1 regular-sized, coarsely chopped onion; adding the wine marinade and 1½ cups of water. Add 1 beef bouillon cube, some garlic salt, a bay leaf, a pinch of thyme, salt and pepper. Cover and simmer for 1½ hours.

While these ingredients are simmering, scrub about 5 new potatoes, paring out any eyes or rough or bad spots. Peel about half a dozen carrots and also 6 or 8 small boiling onions. (These onions often come in a string sack in your grocery store.) Slice the potatoes in half and the carrots in fourths.

When ½ hour is over, throw in the potatoes, onions, and carrots, and continue to simmer for about an hour, testing the vegetables occasionally with a fork for tenderness. You may need to add more water during this hour. The meat will be very tender; no need to worry about it.

Optional: about 15 minutes before the cooking is over, add 1 8-ounce can of tomatoes, undrained. You can add or substract just about any vegetable you want to the stew.

Breaded Cube Steak / Level 2

These small, tenderized steaks can be made interesting. Arrange in a row a paper towel, a cereal bowl, and another paper towel. On the first towel place a layer of flour, crack 1 egg into the bowl and stir it vigorously with a fork, and on the other paper towel make a layer of bread crumbs. Sprinkle parmesan cheese on the crumbs and mix with a fork or your fingers. Your assembly line for breading the steaks is now ready. First dip a steak in flour, making sure it is well-floured. Now immerse it in the egg. (1 egg is enough for 2 small steaks.) Then coat it in the crumb and cheese mixture, getting as much of the mixture as possible to stick to the steak.

Cover the bottom of a frying pan with oil and warm over medium heat until it sizzles. Now fry the steaks for 3 minutes a side, or slightly less if a fork test indicates that the batter is forming too hard a crust. This is a very distant—and very economical—cousin of the cordon bleu.

Pan-Broiled Steak / Level 2

Americans are engaged in a never ending love affair with the steak. Even skyrocketing beef prices do not seem to diminish our ardor for the steak, particularly the charcoal broiled one. True broiling, however, is a dangerous and tricky business when you cannot see, and I recommend that you do not try it. At all.

There is another way, however. Just follow these directions for pan-broiling, and you will be surprised and pleased by the result.

A sirloin, porterhouse, or del Monaco is a good cut to choose. It should be from ¾ to 1¼-inch thick, and it is important that the steak be cut evenly, so that it will broil evenly throughout.

Marinating: this is optional, but tends to improve the flavor. Smear about a teaspoon of oil and vinegar on each side of the steak 15 minutes before broiling. Commercial Italian salad dressing is ideal for a marinade.

Use a heavy, cast-iron frying pan. Before you start, put a dab of bacon fat in the pan and spread it around. The bacon fat is not to grease the pan, it serves as a temperature indicator. Now preheat the pan at a little below medium heat for about 15 minutes. When the pan is hot enough, the bacon fat will begin to smoke, and this you can smell. You may salt the bottom of the pan lightly if you like your steak salted; it also helps to prevent the steak from sticking to the pan. Just before you place the steak in the pan, turn the heat up to medium-high to compensate for the coldness of the steak when it first hits the pan. Put the steak in the pan and turn the heat back down to medium.

If the steak is ¾-inch thick, pan broil it for 4 minutes on each side. Give a 1¼-inch thick steak a little better than 6 minutes per side. This produces a medium-rare steak.

Pan-broiling has a unique advantage; it sears the bottom of the steak so that the juices do not run out. If broiled in the conventional manner where the broiler flame comes from above, the juices can run out below. By the second time you prepare a steak in this way, it will seem almost second nature.

Beef Stroganoff / Level 3

For this preparation, a Level 3 that turns out to be not so exotic after all, you will need dried dill weed. Do not buy dill seed by mistake. Dill weed can be bought in a small bottle in the spice section of your supermarket. It is a good addition to red and yellow vegetables—tomatoes, beets, yellow summer squash, for instance—so it is not extravagant to invest in it for your spice and herb collection.

Freeze 1 pound of round steak. This is to make it easier to cut into small very thin slices, practically slivering it. Sear the slivered steak quickly in a little shortening over medium heat. Dump them into a pot. Now chop 1 yellow onion and sauté it in the frying pan with the shortening, being sure to add more shortening. Put the onion in the pot too, and add ¾ cup of tomato juice, 1 broken bay leaf, a little salt, pepper, and paprika, and a dash of Tabasco sauce (optional). If this seems too dry, add a little water. Simmer the mix for 30 minutes covered, or until the meat is tender but not falling apart. Sample the meat for tenderness and do not overcook. In a cup blend 2 tablespoons flour and 2 tablespoons water. Stir this bit by bit into the mix to thicken it as you desire. Last add 1 small can of mushrooms, drained; or about a ½ dozen fresh mushrooms, sautéed and halved; 1 small 8-ounce container of sour cream; and stir in a little less than ½ teaspoon of dill weed. Bring to a simmer again. Serve over rice. Serves 3 or 4.

Creamed Chicken Pie / Level 2

Here is another uncomplicated company dinner dish-in-one. You begin with a leftover roasted chicken; strip off most of its meat and slice into small chunks. Set the chicken aside.

You will need a double boiler to make the cream sauce. In the top of the boiler place 6 tablespoons or about half a stick of butter. Let it melt slowly, and add 6 teaspoons of flour, 1 teaspoon at a time. While you are doing this, warm 2 cups of milk in a separate pan. Now add the warm milk and stir vigorously with a fork—better still, use a wire whisk if you have one—until the sauce thickens. Add salt and pepper to taste, and a pinch of nutmeg. Now cook over lowered heat in the top of the boiler for 15 to 20 minutes to rid the sauce of the raw taste of the flour.

Now place the chicken chunks in a round oven dish. (A soufflé dish, about 9 inches in diameter and 4 inches deep would be ideal.) Pour the sauce over the chicken, and stir in 1 small can of small peas. For topping use about half a dozen of the biscuits that come ready-made in a cardboard tube. Place in the oven at the temperature indicated for the biscuits, and bake for 10 to 12 minutes.

Baked Chicken / Level 2

There are three simple things you can do to chicken in the oven: roast it, bake it with batter, bake it without batter.

This is the without-batter oven chicken. Remember that you need to add something for interesting flavor, plus a little moisture, and that you cook it covered to keep it moist.

Use a flat-bottomed glass or metal dish, preferably about 3 inches deep. Butter it. You can use a whole, cut-up chicken or limit it to one kind of chicken part.

For instance: rinse chicken thighs in cold water and arrange them, touching on the bottom of the dish. Sprinkle them with a pinch of basil and an envelope of dried onion soup mix. Sprinkle 2 or 3 tablespoons of water on to the soup mix. Now spoon 1 can of cream of chicken soup evenly over the chicken. You can use cream of mushroom or cream of celery if you wish. Cover with aluminum foil and bake in a 325° oven for 1½ hours.

Any kind of chicken goes well with rice or flat noodles.

For an Italian variant: sprinkle an envelope of spaghetti sauce mix over the chicken. Drain 1 can of tomatoes, saving the juice to drink or add to tomato soup. Using a serrated knife, cut the tomatoes up into chunks in the can. Add ¾ cup of white wine. Cover and cook as before.

Almost Fried Chicken / Level 2

Real southern fried chicken done in a skillet on top of the stove is very messy and is quite difficult to do nonvisually, particularly if an entire cut-up chicken with all its different-sized parts is used. Here is a solution that is not merely viable but juicy and crisp.

Put 1 cup of flour (biscuit flour is best) into a plastic bag (paper works too, but is messier). Shake in some salt, pepper, garlic powder, onion salt. Now put half a stick of margarine and a heaping serving spoon of vegetable shortening into a large baking dish and place it in an oven preheated to 425°. Shake up 6 chicken breasts one by one in the plastic bag until they are well-coated. Obviously you could use the thighs or wings instead, or a whole chicken.

With your oven mitts, open the oven door cautiously and slide out the rack on which you set the oven dish. Place the chicken breasts top side up and cook them for about 25 minutes. Open the oven and again, using oven mitts, slide out the rack holding the oven dish. Using tongs or a large fork, turn the chicken breasts over and let them roast for another 25 minutes. If the final product is not crispy enough (make sure you have used plenty of batter) let the chicken bake 5 minutes more on each side. Just tell 'em you got the recipe from the Colonel.

Roast Stuffed Chicken / Level 2

In spite of today's high prices, chicken is still one of the best bargains to be had at the meat counter. Better still, there is nothing to waste.

Remove the giblets and neck from the cavity of the whole roaster chicken you have bought. Rinse the chicken. Rub the chicken well with vegetable oil; this helps to hold in the juices and make some of the skin crisp. Set the chicken on a rack in a roasting pan and pour 2 cups of water into the pan. The chicken will then steam as it roasts, which helps to keep the meat, particularly the breast portions, from becoming dry. Place in an oven preheated to 450°, reduce the temperature immediately to 350°, and roast for 20 minutes per pound. That's all there is to it.

Stuffing: commercial stuffing mixes are reasonably priced and almost absurdly simple to use. Have someone read the directions on the package; usually you will need to add only butter and hot water. You may wish to add the giblets and some mushrooms, sautéed, before you stuff the chicken.

If any of the chicken is leftover, you can use it for chicken salad, chicken sandwiches, or chicken pie (see the next preparation). And don't throw away the bones or the chicken neck; from them you can make a good chicken soup, directions for which are on page 69.

Fried Liver / Level 2

I have never met anyone who is neutral about liver. Either you like it a lot, or you can't stand it. First choice for this preparation is calf's liver, second, baby beef, and adult beef a poor third. Pork liver is for cats. A liver does not freeze or save well, so buy only enough for one meal.

Put some flour on a paper plate and flour both sides of the liver. You can fold up the paper plate and throw it away without any mess. Melt a generous amount of butter, at least 1 tablespoon, in a frying pan over medium-low heat. Place the liver in the pan and immediately reduce the heat to very low. Fry for 4 minutes, then turn over and fry for 3 minutes. Use a timer, because it is important not to overcook.

If you like liver and onions—I know I do—they go best cooked in bacon fat. Fry 5 or 6 strips of bacon, remove the bacon from the pan and drain on a paper towel, and then fry the onions. Cut 3 or 4 slices from an onion, and then punch the slices apart into rings. Fry the onions until they begin to turn soft, then push them to both sides of the pan and fry the liver as above.

Chicken livers should be fried in butter or little oil, not bacon fat. These small livers take less than a minute each side over low heat.

Pork Chops / Level 2

I like to treat myself to a thick pork chop for this preparation, not the thinner and less expensive chops that are sometimes called breakfast pork chops.

Heat your frying pan for 3 or 4 minutes over medium heat. Now the pan is good and hot. Brown the chops for 3 or 4 minutes on each side, turning with a large fork. Reduce the flame to very low.

These thick chops have already fried for 8 minutes or so. Now that you have turned the heat down, cook them for 20 minutes more on each side, covered.

It is essential to keep pork chops from drying out if you are frying them. My two favorite ways:

1. Pour in a little cheap red wine, or wine and water. Keep an attentive ear to the chops as they cook, and add more liquid if you hear them drying out.

2. Add half a can of cream of mushroom soup on top of the chops, undiluted, and the other half when you turn the chops over.

Pork Chop and Corn Oven Dish / Level 2

These chops do not require previous browning. Use the thinner, cheaper breakfast chops. You need a pan or shallow baking dish large enough for six chops and the extras. (Note: a metal pan should be slightly greased to prevent sticking.) Mix together 1 can (15 ounces) of cream-style corn, half a chopped onion, 1 egg fork-beaten, and 2 slices of crumbled toast. Place the pork chops on the bottom of the pan and moisten them with a little milk. Pile the stuffing mix on top of them. Cover the pan with a lid or aluminum foil. Bake at 325° for about 2 hours. (Careful: sharp bones may result when the meat falls off them. Best serve with a large cooking spoon; a fork won't lift the chops.)

I test-cooked this dish for a friend from Houston who, incredibly enough, had never in his life eaten corn. He told me he liked the corn. I liked the chops, too.

Roasts / Level 2

Since you cannot use a meat thermometer, you need a table to tell you how long per pound to roast different meats. Here it is: these times are approximate. The roasting temperature for all meats is 325°.

Beef: rare, a little less than ½ hour per pound; medium, just over ½ hour per pound; well done, ¾ hour per pound.

Fresh ham: ½ hour per pound.

Pork loin: 1 hour per pound.

Leg of lamb: ½ hour per pound.

Boned rolled shoulder of lamb: ¾ hour per pound.

Veal: Leg, just under ½ hour per pound; loin, just over ½ hour per pound; boned rolled shoulder, just under ¾ hour per pound.

You need to use a rack with all boneless roasts. When cooking a bone-in roast, place the bone side down.

German Sauerbraten / Level 2

Sauerbraten is a traditional marinated beef dish. Much German beef is tough, rarely of steak quality. So this is a preparation that allows us to make use of cheaper roast cuts.

My food preparation avoids the pitfalls of most sauerbraten recipes you may find. It does not use any vinegar; the cheap wine does the job by itself. It does not call for ginger snaps or any other sweetener. Why should the meat sit in a muck of disintegrated cookies? It does, on the other hand, demand that you marinate the beef for four days minimum rather than just a few hours or overnight.

In a large roasting pan, combine the following to make the marinade: 1 quart of cheap burgundy, 1½ tablespoons of dried onion flakes, 2 bay leaves, 6 cloves, 1 teaspoon of poultry seasoning, ½ teaspoon of black pepper, 1 teaspoon garlic salt, 1½ teaspoons of tarragon leaves (essential). Simmer a few minutes to let ingredients dissolve and mix. Then place a 2-pound roast—chuck, pot, or arm roast—in the mixture. Add water to immerse the meat if necessary. Let it marinate in the refrigerator for 4 days. Then simmer on the stove for 2 to 3 hours, until the meat falls apart at the poke of a fork. Use a slotted spoon to lift and drain chunks of sauerbraten, and serve over rice. I like to make a rice mixture, adding brown and/or wild rice to flavor the white rice.

Fried Fish / Level 2

The commonest frozen fish seem to be codfish, haddock, ocean perch, flounder, and catfish.

Fish taste best if they are cooked when just barely thawed and not warmed through to room temperature. This takes 1 to 2 hours at room temperature or about 8 hours in the refrigerator.

The fish should be breaded. Cover it well on both sides with flour seasoned with salt and pepper. If you want a thicker batter, then dip the fish into a fork-beaten egg and then again in the flour or corn meal. Fry the fish in about ¼ inch of oil. You can judge the amount by listening as you pour it into the pan; and then brushing the bottom of the pan with your fingers to discover how much oil you can splash around.

Fry the fish for 4 to 8 minutes on each side, over medium heat. How long they need to fry depends entirely on the thickness of each piece, so you must try to decide whether each piece is relatively thin or relatively thick.

You can also deep-fry the fish by immersing it in hot oil and frying for 5 to 8 minutes, no turning necessary. Tartar sauce, of course, is the traditional sauce for fried white fish.

Oven Fish Fillets / Level 2

For many of us, frozen is just the way that fish come. But if you are a fisherman or have a fish market in your town, so much the better. You can treat almost any kind of ordinary fish this way. Thaw the fish, but not completely. Place a sheet of aluminum foil in a shallow baking pan or on a cookie sheet. Now lay down the fillets, lightly salted and peppered if you wish, side by side. You can add any kind of herbs or spices that you wish, such as basil, parsley, or paprika. You can add a little chopped onion or bell pepper, or a very thin slice of cheese. Especially with rather thin fillets, this helps retain the moisture of the fish.

Bake in a preheated 425° oven for about 20 minutes. It depends on the thickness of the fillets. My fish consultant hedged when I asked him to be more specific. Besides, he is down by the brook right now. 15 or 20 minutes is average. The best way to judge is by smell. Fork testing helps some. You may not wish to eat the fillets with tartar sauce; it goes better with the less subtle taste of pan-fried fish.

Try this sauce: before putting the fillets in the oven, prepare this sauce in a small saucepan. For one portion of fish, use 2 tablespoons of melted butter and 2 teaspoons of concentrated lemon juice. Melt the butter over a low flame, tipping the pan over the flame so that the butter will not burn. Add only one of the following: a pinch, which is about ⅛ teaspoon, of basil, dill weed, dried parsley, garlic salt or paprika. Dribble this sauce onto the fillets before placing them into the oven.

Quiche / Level 2

You don't have to be a pastry cook to make this quiche. The preparation uses a ready-made frozen pie crust.

Combine: 1 tablespoon of flour, 3 tablespoons of milk, 4 tablespoons of mayonnaise, and 1 egg. These should be well-mixed so use a wire whisk if you have one.

Now you need to separate an egg in order to obtain the egg white for coating the pie shell. Crack 1 cold egg on the rim of the mixing bowl, and hold it over a cup. If you have one, use an egg separator to separate the yolk and the white. Otherwise, hold it from beneath with your left hand and finish pulling the shell apart with your right; the raw egg will slide into the palm of your left hand. Let the white run through your fingers into the cup, and add the yolk to the mixture in the bowl. Now pour the white into the pie shell, and spread it well around the bottom sides and rim. Pour the excess white into the mixing bowl. Grate ½ cup or more of Swiss cheese and add to the bowl. Also add a cup or more of ham, cut into rather small pieces. You can add a small can of mushrooms, drained, if you wish. Or, if you do not have the ham, you can make the quiche with 2 small cans or 1 medium-sized can of mushrooms instead.

Stir the ingredients and fill the pie shell, spreading them evenly. Bake in a 350° oven for 45 minutes. Serves 4 or 5.

Stuffed Bell Peppers / Level 2

This is a good one to play with, because so many different fillings are possible.

Cut out the stem ends of as many bell peppers as you are preparing. Remove the core, seeds, and the fibrous strips along the walls with a paring knife. You can save the caps to use in a salad, if you wish.

Some fillings: leftover spaghetti, ground beef with rice, canned Spanish rice, macaroni and cheese. Whatever filling you choose should best be composed of some sort of meat, some sort of starch, and a sauce. Diced leftover chicken is a good ingredient.

Parboil the pepper cases for 5 minutes, drain them, and stand them in a fairly deep baking dish. Spoon in the filling mixture until the peppers are full but not heaping.

Bake peppers at 350°, uncovered, for 20 minutes. Baste with tomato sauce, sprinkle with cheese; bake 10 minutes longer.

Eggs Benedict / Level 3

Start with the hollandaise sauce mix. The kind of sauce mix I use makes ¾ cup per envelope, which is enough for 2 servings. Follow the envelope directions that were read to you, being sure to mix with cold water at first. When the sauce has thickened, which you can tell by the way it drips from your spoon, move the saucepan to the back of the stove. A ¾-inch slice of ham or Canadian bacon can have been warming in a small frying pan all along, because the timing for it is not crucial.

Put half an English muffin in the toaster. While it is toasting, bring 2 inches of water in another small saucepan to a boil. When the muffin pops up, turn off the heat under the boiling water, and crack an egg into the water. Turn on the heat again and let the egg poach for about 2 minutes, which gives you enough time to butter the muffin and place it on the full-sized dinner plate. Turn off the boiling water. Place the ham slice on the buttered muffin. Lift the poached egg out with a slotted spoon and place it on the ham. Remember that you will seldom be able to lift all the egg out at once. Spoon the hollandaise sauce over the egg. Use a serrated knife and a fork to eat the egg benedict.

Eggplant Parmesan / Level 3

This is an excellent company meal. I call it Level 3 simply because it takes patience to make and you must be careful to slice the eggplant evenly.

Arrange 3 shallow bowls from left to right. Put flour in the first; 3 or 4 beaten eggs and a little milk in the next; and bread crumbs in the third. Wash the eggplant, and slice it into thin, even slices (¼ to ⅜ inch). Do not peel. Flour each piece well, then dip in the eggs and bread crumbs. Stack the slices on a plate as you do so.

Now deep-fry the slices. Here's how: pour cooking oil about ¼-inch deep into a large cast-iron skillet. Heat over medium flame until the oil sizzles, then reduce the flame to low, and the oil will continue to sizzle but not smoke. Using a fork or tongs, place 4 or 5 slices in the oil in a circle. They need to deep-fry a couple of minutes on each side until, using a fork, you can feel that the batter is turning crusty and the eggplant is tender. Proceed around the circle in the order you put the slices into the pan, and of course they will finish cooking in the same order. Lift them out of the pan and drain them on several layers of paper towel. Now you are ready to fry 4 or 5 more slices, but you will probably have to add some more oil each time.

I find that to fry all of a medium-sized eggplant is too much. Eggplants do not freeze and will spoil very quickly; so if you cannot fry up the rest within 48 hours, throw it away.

To finish building the casserole, you need 20 to 24 ounces of tomato sauce, a ½ pound of fresh mushrooms—you can cheat and substitute canned ones, and about 8 ounces each of grated parmesan and mozarella cheese. Slice the mushrooms in half and sauté them. Layer all those ingredients with the eggplant in a deep casserole dish, finishing with a layer of mozarella cheese. As you layer, sprinkle in a ½ teaspoon of oregano, a pinch at a time.

About 3 or 4 layers will result. Bake in a medium 350° oven for 30 minutes, until hot and bubbly. Ideal with a tossed salad and chilled wine.

Steak and Mushroom Pie / Level 2

This dish has a family resemblance to the creamed chicken pie, and is no more difficult to prepare. I have misled you somewhat with the title, though, because I suggest you use stew meat instead of steak to save money. Buy 1 pound of stew meat, trimmed and cut, at the supermarket. Slice the larger pieces into hearty bite-sized chunks. Put them in a paper bag with flour, salt, and pepper and shake to coat the pieces. Brown them in a deep skillet for about 10 minutes, using 5 tablespoons of oil. Stir the meat while it is browning. Now add 3 cups of hot water in which 6 beef bouillon cubes have been dissolved. Cover and simmer for about 1½ hours. Check after an hour to make sure that the water has not boiled too low.

While the meat is cooking, take 1 pound of fresh mushrooms and wash well. Do this by rinsing them thoroughly first. Then rub the mushroom caps lightly across a plastic scrubber. Cut them in half. Melt half a stick of butter or margarine and sauté the mushrooms. Turn them with a fork. This will take about 10 minutes over low heat, and reduce the mushrooms considerably in volume. When the meat is finished cooking, dump the mushrooms and butter into the skillet. Mix 3 tablespoons of water with 3 tablespoons of flour in a cup. Stir this into the skillet until reaching the thickness of gravy you desire. If you want a rather thick gravy, you can judge its thickness by the way it drips from your spoon. Next pour the contents of the skillet into a deep oven dish, using oven mitts for safety. Make a topping of ready-made biscuits. Bake in the oven for the time and temperature recommended for the biscuits.

Spaghetti Sauce / Level 2

Brown 1 pound of ground beef and drain the grease, if there is any. Chop and add 1 bell pepper and 1 yellow onion. Flavor with oregano, garlic salt, and coarse pepper, starting with ½ teaspoon oregano and garlic salt and ¼ teaspoon pepper and adding more if necessary. Add 2 15-ounce cans of tomato sauce and 1 small can of tomato paste. You can add 1 chopped tomato, fresh or canned. Add 1 can of mushrooms drained. Don't skip this last ingredient: a ½ cup of red wine, preferably burgundy. Simmer for about 20 minutes while you are cooking the spaghetti and getting the parmesan cheese out of the cupboard.

Now that you have served the spaghetti and the sauce, you need a tip about how to eat it. Some people cut up their spaghetti. This is not merely an affront to Italian food, however, it makes it even harder for blind people to eat spaghetti. Instead, do it the traditional way. Holding a soup spoon in your left hand, vertical to, and touching, the plate. Slide your fork at a right angle through the spaghetti and sauce toward the spoon. Now twist the fork in the bowl of the spoon so that the spaghetti and sauce wraps around the fork. Open your mouth wide: you'll taste the real thing.

Brown Gravy / Level 2

Gravy goes well on a roast or stew of any sort, or on the potatoes that accompany it.

The basic proportions for one cup of brown gravy are: for one cup of liquid consisting of meat drippings and water, two tablespoons of fat (not counting any fat that may be in the liquid) and two tablespoons of flour. For liquid, you should start with whatever is in the roasting pan when the meat is finished. Pour those drippings into a small saucepan and from the saucepan into a measuring cup to judge the amount. Then back into the saucepan. Add some more fat. Just guess at how much fat might be in the drippings; it doesn't matter that much. Was it a fatty cut of roast? You can use leftover bacon fat, but solid vegetable shortening seems to be best.

If, say, you wanted to make 2 cups of gravy, subtract the ¾ cup of drippings you measured, and pour 1¼ cups of cold water into a bowl. Cold, because you can stir flour into it without it getting lumpy. Stir in 3½ tablespoons flour, the right proportion for this example. Add it to the saucepan slowly, stiring over low heat. Judge the thickness you want by letting the gravy drip from the spoon you are stirring with. Add more water if the gravy gets too thick.

If there was not enough meat flavoring, add 2 beef bouillon cubes. You may want to add a teaspoon of commercial gravy-maker, which comes in a small bottle among the other condiments at the supermarket. You can also add any of the following: salt, pepper, garlic salt, dried onion flakes, dried parsley.

Instead of cold water, you can use milk to make a creamier gravy.

Lasagna / Level 3

This Level 3 preparation takes 2½ hours to make. The ingredients cost between seven and eight dollars, but it makes a good dinner for 6.

Take a large, deep skillet and crumble 1 pound of ground beef into it. Brown it slowly over low flame. While it is browning, peel and chop ½ an onion. Add the onion to the skillet. Continue to brown. Sprinkle in ½ teaspoon each of oregano and garlic powder. Or 1 teaspoon of garlic salt.

Wash and trim ½ pound of fresh mushrooms. Do this by placing them in a sieve and running cold water over them, and running their caps lightly over a plastic scrubber. Trim off the tough part of the stems and slice the mushrooms in two. Open a space in the center of the skillet and put ⅓ of a stick of margarine in it to melt. Add the split mushrooms and simmer them.

While this is happening, follow the directions on a box of lasagna noodles that have been read to you. The noodles must be boiled in a large enough pan or else they will stick together.

Grate 8 ounces of mozarella cheese onto a large cutting board. Afterwards the noodles should be done. Drain them in the sieve, and run cold water on them so you can handle them. You are going to need cottage cheese and parmesan cheese as well.

Now you are ready to build the lasagna. Use a rectangular glass dish. Mine is 13 x 9 x 2 inches and is also good for baking enchiladas.

My box of noodles had twelve of them in it, which makes three convenient layers. Lay down four noodles. Scoop the entire contents of the skillet onto them with a slotted spoon. Pour about 16 ounces of your favorite tomato sauce over it, smoothing and leveling the layer with the back of the spoon.

Put down another layer of noodles. Scoop on 8 to 12 ounces of cottage cheese. I use small curd and do not try to drain it. Sprinkle on a double handful of the loose, grated mozarella. Now comes the third layer of noodles. Add the rest of the mozarella and a double handful of parmesan cheese. Again smooth and even out the layer with the back of the spoon. Now heat the lasagna, uncovered, in a 350° oven for 30 minutes.

This is one of those dishes that taste even better when reheated the second time around. And you can freeze the leftovers if you wish. It is also one of those dishes that people will find hard to believe a blind cook has successfully prepared.

Cover the lasagna dish with aluminum foil when you refrigerate the leftovers, and leave the foil on when reheating. If you want to reheat just one portion, scoop it into a small oven dish and pour some more tomato sauce over it to keep it moist.

Baking

Introductory Note

Frequent baking calls for accurate measuring and timing greatly facilitated by judgments based on eyesight. This is particularly true of complicated cakes made from scratch and yeast-rising breads. The basic items described here will allow you to estimate what recipes from traditional cookbooks you can attempt. The many prepackaged mixes available today cost more than ingredients bought separately, of course, but they will allow you to bake many things that might otherwise be beyond your skills level.

Refrigerator Biscuits and Cookies / Level 1

Just have someone read the directions printed on the biscuit or cookie tube, and then keep these points in mind:

1. It is important that the oven be fully preheated before you put the biscuits in, because precise time and temperature is important.

2. Bake the biscuits only as long as the minimum time limit given. That is, if the container specifies 8 to 10 minutes, bake for only 8 minutes. They will continue to bake a little while cooling.

3. Once you open a tube of biscuits, bake all of them at once. The unbaked biscuit dough will not keep.

4. Biscuits usually come precut, cookies usually do not. There are directions for cutting the cookie dough on the container, but remember this: it is very important to cut the cookies the same size for evenness in baking, but it is harder to do so than you may think. Feel the individual cookies carefully after you have arranged them on the baking sheet. With a knife, subtract a little from the ones that are too big and press it onto the ones that are too little. The pieced-together cookies will not break apart.

Oatmeal Cookies / Level 2

Drop cookies are the simplest kind, because you just spoon the dough onto the cookie sheet. I'll just give you the procedure for oatmeal and chocolate chip cookies. Once you know how to make drop cookies you can handle all sorts of cookie preparations found in other cookbooks.

Melt ¾ cup or 1½ sticks of butter or margarine in a medium skillet over very low heat. Then stir in 2½ cups of uncooked oatmeal. Stir constantly and cook for 5 minutes. If the butter starts to smell at all scorched, try to turn the heat down even lower. At the end of the 5 minutes, turn off the heat.

Break 1 egg into a mixing bowl and add 1 teaspoon of vanilla. Stir with a fork. Add 1 cup of brown sugar and stir vigorously until this is thoroughly and smoothly mixed.

In another bowl, sift ½ cup of all-purpose flour, 1 teaspoon of cinnamon, and ½ teaspoon of baking soda. Add these to the sugar mixture and again blend thoroughly with a fork. Now add in the oatmeal and butter mixture and blend them with a fork. You are probably wondering whether the batter will be moist enough. It will be.

Now set the oven at 375° and let it preheat thoroughly while you are dropping the cookies. Drop the cookies, 1 rounded teaspoon each, in rows of three on two ungreased cookie sheets. Bake for 10 minutes.

Chocolate Chip Cookies / Level 2

In a large mixing bowl, combine these wet or soft ingredients thoroughly with a fork: 2 eggs, 1 teaspoon vanilla, 1 cup (that's one stick) of soft butter or margarine. Now add 1 teaspoon of baking soda and 2¼ cups of ordinary flour and mix them in very thoroughly with the fork. Add ¾ cup of brown sugar, and 8 ounces of chocolate chips. Again, mix very thoroughly with a fork, feeling with your hand to make sure that all the chips are distributed evenly. You may add about a cup of chopped nuts if you like.

Set the oven at 375° and let it preheat while you drop the cookies. Drop them a heaping teaspoon at a time on an ungreased cookie sheet, three to a row. Bake for 9 minutes. This makes about 40 cookies.

Cornbread / Level 2

Every package of corn meal has directions for cornbread on it. Have someone read them to you. There are slight variations from package to package.

Keep these things in mind while preparing the cornbread: you can omit the sugar, particularly if you are going to eat the cornbread with something sweet, such as syrup or honey. You can use cooking oil instead of solid shortening. It mixes more easily. Mix the wet ingredients first, then add the dry ones. Grease the pan well. Lots of batter will stick to the bowl. Hold it from beneath with one hand, resting the bottom of the upturned bowl against your chest. Holding a spoon in the other hand, you can then scrape out the remaining batter. With the bottom of the spoon, spread the batter out evenly in the pan.

That's it. This is an easy Level 2.

Banana Bread / Level 2

You'll need 2 very ripe bananas—ripe enough to squash easily with a fork. Start with ⅔ cup of white sugar, ⅓ cup of brown sugar, and ⅓ cup of shortening. Cut them together with a fork. Now mix in the following ingredients also with a fork without resorting to a food-beater: 3 eggs, 1¾ cups of flour, 2¾ teaspoons of baking powder, ¼ teaspoon of salt, 1 teaspoon each of cinnamon, nutmeg and vanilla, and ½ cup of chopped pecans (optional).

Now slice in the 2 ripe bananas and blend thoroughly with a fork. Grease a 9 x 9 metal baking dish or a breadloaf pan. Bake in a 325° oven for about 1 hour; you can use the toothpick or broom straw method to test for doneness.

Cake Mixes / Level 3

These directions apply to any standard box cake mix. Be sure to have someone read the back of the package to you, because you need to know individual baking times and temperatures, as well as any special direction that may be necessary.

Place any ingredients you may need to add to the mix into a large bowl before adding the mix itself. Water, eggs, and oil are common ingredients. Then add the mix and blend it with a fork until you can feel that all the large, powdery lumps are gone. But the batter is still far from sufficiently mixed. Use a hand-turned food mixer to beat the batter. It will often say on the package how many strokes are recommended. If it does not, 400 is what I recommend. This is a boring job, and your arm will get tired. I beat it 100 strokes at a time and rest a little in between. I'm in no hurry.

Grease and flour whatever baking pans you are going to use: a glass dish, 2 8-inch or 9-inch round pans, or a cake mold. I like to use a nonstick cake mold, because it saves me the tricky work of layering. Spread butter on the inside of the pans with your fingers, and then put in about a tablespoon of ordinary flour. Tip the pan almost vertically and rotate it, shaking it as you do so. Then dump out the flour that did not stick.

Pour in the batter, using a spoon to scrape the bowl clean. Bake in a preheated oven for the time directed, but do not rely on your timer alone. You should use the time-honored technique of the broomstraw as well. Plunge a clean broomstraw into the cake. If it comes out clean, the cake is done. And not until then.

Let the cake cool to room temperature before trying to remove it from the pan. Some pans have a loosening device that you turn to make sure the layer is not sticking. Place a plastic dinner plate or cake dish upside down over the layer. Invert it and knock it sharply on the counter or table. The pan should lift free, leaving the layer intact.

Frosting. I use ready-made frosting that comes in a can. A standard 1-pound can is enough for 2 whole cakes. Open the can and place it in a saucepan that has about 2 inches of water in it. Turn on the heat and let the water boil over low heat until the frosting becomes quite fluid. You can feel this by stirring it with a teaspoon. Now place the saucepan right next to the cake plate and spoon the frosting out of the can teaspoon by teaspoon onto the cake. Be sure to drip frosting along the sides.

Making a Pie / Level 2

You could call this the patty-cake method of pie-making, since it avoids the very difficult process of rolling out the pie crust.

Instead, you make it in the pie pan itself, with no rolling pin at all.

Measure 1½ cups of ordinary flour into a pie pan or glass pie dish (ungreased). Spread it over the bottom of the pan. Now sprinkle in 1½ teaspoons of sugar and 2 tablespoons of milk. Add a ½ cup of salad oil.

Mix the dough thoroughly with your fingers, pinching all the lumps to blend the flour in. Now press the dough evenly along the sides and bottom of the pan. You will be surprised how easy this is.

Fruit fillings. The simplest are the pie apples or cherries bought in a can or jar, or simply applesauce. You can add cinnamon to the applesauce. If you use fresh fruit, such as sliced apples or peaches, use about a ½ cup of sugar, adding just enough water to the sugar to dissolve it into syrup. Bake fresh fruit pies at 350° for 50 minutes.

Bake other pies for 45 minutes in a preheated, 400° oven. Place a cookie sheet underneath them to catch any drippings.

Appendix

For easy reference I have here grouped the food preparations into Levels 1, 2 and 3.

Level 1

Breakfast
Cold cereal
Making toast
Scramble-fried eggs
Hard-boiled eggs
Breakfast sausage, links or patties
Oven-fried bacon

Lunch
Hot dogs
Sandwiches

Vegetables
Rice
Coleslaw
Salad dressing
Baked potatoes

Baking
Refrigerator biscuits and cookies

Level 2

Breakfast

Hot cereal
Scrambled eggs
Soft-boiled eggs
Fried eggs, sunnyside up
The unflippable fried egg
Fried eggs easy over
Poached eggs
The basic omelette
Pan-fried bacon
Pancakes
Rice pudding

Lunch

Hot dogs and bacon
Pigs in blankets
Grilled cheese sandwich
Reuben sandwich
Hamburgers
Macaroni salad
Hearty bean soup
Split pea soup
Chicken soup

Vegetables

Bean salad
Acorn squash
Baked summer squash with cheese
Creamed onions
Guacamole
American fries
German fried potatoes
Hash brown potatoes
Scalloped potatoes
Cold potato salad
German style potato salad

Dinner

Cheese and meat casseroles
Zucchini casserole
Meat loaf
Fried eggs on canned meat
Chili for Yankees
Breaded cube steak
Pan-broiled steak
Creamed chicken pie
Baked chicken
Almost fried chicken
Roast stuffed chicken
Fried liver
Pork chops
Pork chop and corn oven dish

Roasts

German sauerbraten
Fried fish
Oven fish fillets
Quiche
Stuffed bell peppers
Steak and mushroom pie
Spaghetti sauce
Brown gravy

Baking

Oatmeal cookies
Chocolate chip cookies
Cornbread
Banana bread
Making a pie

Level 3

Lunch

Devilled eggs
Onion cheese potato cakes

Baking

Cake mixes

Dinner

Tamale pie
Easy enchiladas
Beef stew, marinated
Beef stroganoff
Eggs benedict
Eggplant parmesan
Lasagna